THE RE-CENTER METHOD NATURAL DIET

HOLIDAY & CHRISTMAS DESSERTS

Celebrate the Joy of Feasting

International Recipes from 7 Continents
For All Holidays

Hareldau Argyle King

Also Available from Refinement Publishing & Media

Quotes to Habits
Remember

Hareldau Argyle King

The Re-center Method
Natural Diet
Hareldau Argyle King

The Re-center Method
Natural Diet Cookbook
Hareldau Argyle King

The Re-center Method
Natural Diet Saladbook
Hareldau Argyle King

The Re-center Method
Natural Diet Soupbook
Hareldau Argyle King

© Copyright November 2023

by Refinement Publishing & Media

Published by Refinement Publishing &Media - All rights reserved.

Web site: www.beingelevatedlifestyle.com Email: support@beingelevatedlifestyle.com

As with all exercises and dietary programs, you should get your doctor's approval before beginning. The information here is to help you make an informed decision about your health.

This book is not intended as a substitute for any treatment that may have been prescribed by your doctor. The reader should regularly consult a doctor in matters about his/her health and particularly concerning any symptoms that may require diagnosis or medical attention.

This book is intended as a reference manual and not a medical manual. The exercises and dietary programs in the book are not intended as a substitute for any exercise routine or dietary regimen that may have been prescribed by your doctor.

Copyright © 2023 by Refinement Publishing &Media All rights reserved.

All rights reserved. No part of the publication may be reproduced or transmitted in any form or by any means. Without the express written permission of the publisher except for the use of brief quotations in a book review.

The scanning, uploading, and distribution of this book via the internet or any other means without the permission of the publisher are illegal and punishable by law. Please by law Please purchase only authorized electronic editions and do not participate in or encourage electronic piracy of copyrighted materials. Your support of the author's rights is appreciated.

www.beingelevatedlifestyle.com
Ebook ISBN: 978-1-950838-40-0
Hardback ISBN: 978-1-950838-38-7
Paperback ISBN: 978-1-950838-39-4

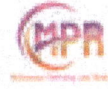

ACKNOWLEDGMENTS

Meals taste better when shared in the community, and even better when shared with stories among family, friends, and colleagues.

I am grateful for every friend, family member, and & passing acquaintance I shared a unique meal, whether the meals were a local dish or an elaborate international meal.

Whether it was served at a dinner party, upscale restaurant, a local diner, or a backyard cookout. In every city I lived, town I passed through, and country every visited I say Thank you.

Your generosity encouraged me to gather & create this collection of recipes from different states and nations.

FOREWORD

Welcome to a tantalizing journey that will take you on a mouthwatering odyssey through the diverse and delectable world of desserts. "The Re-center Method Natural Diet Holiday Desserts" is a culinary masterpiece that celebrates the international tapestry of flavors and traditions, woven together by the common thread of our collective love for all things sweet. In these pages, you will encounter an array of exquisite confections, each representing the unique essence of its place of origin.

As you delve into these tantalizing pages written by my dear friend and sister Hareldau, you will discover that this book is much more than a collection of sweet recipes. It is an invitation to embark on a cultural and culinary voyage that will transport you to the far corners of the globe. The desserts featured within these pages are not mere recipes; they are living testaments to the creativity, artistry, and passion of countless generations.

One of the most extraordinary aspects of desserts is how they provide insight into the complex tapestry of human history and culture. During the holidays, desserts take on a special significance, becoming the sweet embodiment of cultural rituals and cherished memories. From the aromatic gingerbread cookies of Christmas to the vibrant colors of Diwali sweets in India, these delectable treats play a vital role in conveying the spirit of festivities. Desserts have played a vital role in celebrations, rituals, and everyday life for centuries, and they continue to do so today. Whether it'sthe exuberant Carnival season in Brazil, or the refined elegance of afternoon tea in England- desserts have been the sweet accompaniment to our shared human experiences.

They symbolize the togetherness of families, the exchange of love and well-wishes, and the culmination of the year's hard work. The act of preparing and sharing holiday desserts is an expression of hospitality, love, and the continuation of time-honored customs that have been passed down through generations. All in all - desserts bring an extra layer of sweetness to our holidays, forging connections and creating lasting impressions that define the spirit of the season.

Deserts in all its design and beauty provideaprofound connection to nature and spirituality. From the Holy Month of Ramadan celebrated across the Middle East to the colorful traditions of the Day of the Dead in Mexico, deserts play an essential role in grounding these unique and diverse holiday experiences, reminding us of the remarkable interplay between humanity, nature, and the celebration of life's most cherished moments.

This book not only celebrates the diversity of the world's tastiest desserts but also showcases the power of food to bridge gaps, foster connections, and transcend language. The act of sharing a dessert is a universal symbol of hospitality and camaraderie, uniting people in a shared appreciation for the joys of life.

Our hope is that as you explore these recipes and stories, you will be inspired to bring a piece of the world's culture to your own table, savoring the pleasure of not only creating but also sharing these delightful treats with your loved ones.

And lastly, the most important thing to remember about these holiday treats is that while desserts, are a delightful indulgence- they play a surprisingly important role in overall well-being. It can be a source of comfort and nostalgia, bringing us back to cherished memories and creating a sense of happiness and contentment.Moreover, savoring a well-crafted dessert can ignite the senses, providing a moment of mindfulness that allows us to savor the present and momentarily escape the stresses of life.

So, without further ado, let your voyage begin. Our highly esteemed and accomplished author and guide has permitted us to indulge this holiday season – freely!

Immerse yourself in the world of holiday desserts and let your taste buds explore the flavors that have delighted generations. May these pages inspire you to create, share, and savor the sweet moments that life has to offer. We invite you to embark on this scrumptious journey across the continents and, in doing so, discover the world through its most delectable and universal language—food.

Bon appétit!

Natalie Rose Legrand
Founder of The Nourished Leader

DEDICATION

IN HONOR OF
NATALIE LEGRAND

In honor of my friend, Fellow Toastmasters, and humanitarian
Ms. Natalie Legrand lives a life of curiosity, compassion & courage
You are a source of inspiration, excitement & hope
A world traveler, a beautiful spirit, a justice seeker
You constantly keep rising to challenges, in seasons
& times when others buckle,
You wear your heart for divinity, equality, and diversity on your
sleeves. Your friendship is precious to my soul!

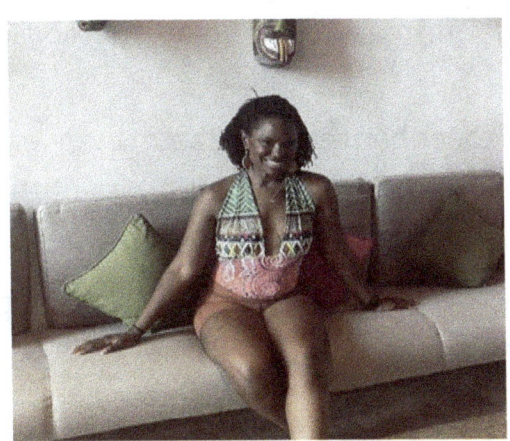

Natalie Rose Legrand

How to Use this Book

This book is a guide to a higher quality of life, through building relationships and varying your food choices. Whether you never had an international meal or friend or whether this is your way of life, there are words of encouragement, new ideas & solutions to enhance your quality of life.

The book is divided into 7 sections. The first section is Pastries Desserts recipes from Africa, Asia, and Australia & Oceania, The Caribbean, Latin America & South America, and North America.

Section 11 consists of Custard recipes, Section 111 Cake recipes, Section 1v Pies & Cobblers recipes Section V Cookies, Section V1 Ice Cream Section V11 Puddings from 7 continents. If you notice a country under a different classification, it may be because some countries may be geographically located in one continent as well as cultural associate with another.

This is not a diet book, a weight loss book, or a meal plan. On your first attempt to prepare these dishes, your meal may or may not look like the photo of the meal in this book.

This book is designed to enhance your taste bud, exposing you to different textures and tastes of food from all the continents of the world. After you would complete this 4-part of series international recipe books+ this bonus book Holidays & Christmas Desserts book, you experience cuisines from 195 countries in 7 continents.

I invite you to get started today. Don't Procrastinate!!

Table of Content

Introduction.
Section 1: Pastries
Africa

South Africa - Koeksisters
Sao Tome Principle- S,onhos de banana (banana dreams)
Cameroon- Chin Chin

Asia

Qatar-Luqaimat
Thailand - KhanomBuang
Myanmar -Mont Lone Yay Paw (Sweet Floating Rice Balls)

Australia & Oceania

French Polynesia.- Firi- Firi
Fiji- Custard Pie
Walls and Futuna -Matafaga

Europe

Ukraine -Medovik
Germany-Willkommen
Switzerland - Swiss Apple Tart

Caribbean

Dominica – Dominica Delight
Grenada- Sweet pastry
Haiti- Pain Patate

South America & Latin America

Honduras- Fried Dough
Brazil-Pastel de Nata
Argentina: Alfajores

North America,

Nashville, Tennessee- Southern Pecan Pie
Victoria, Canada- Nanaimo Bar
Section 11 Custard

Africa
Equatorial Guinea- AsadLeche
Ghana- Milk Tart
Comoros - Vanilla-Ylang Custard

Asia
Israel-Malabi
Mongolia- Boiled Milk Custard Recipe:
Turkmenistan - Gyzgym

Australia & Oceania
Micronesia - Coconut Milk Custard
Vanuatu- Coconut Custard Pie.
New Caledonia -Vanilla Flan

Europe
Austria- Viennese Apple Strudel with Vanilla Sauce
Spain – Flan
Russia - Tvorojniki

Caribbean
Barbados- Bajan Bread Pudding
Cuba - Flan Cubano
St Martin - Caribbean Coconut Flan

South America & Latin America
Peru-Suspiro de Limeña
Guatemala- Rellenitos de Plátano
Aurba- Aruban Coconut Pudding

North America
Alaska- Akutaq (Eskimo Ice Cream)
Mexico Zacatecas- Flan
Calgary, Canada

Section 111 Cakes
Africa
Nigeria - Nigerian Coconut Cake:
Togo - Togolese Banana Cake
Morocco - Orange Cake

Asia

Kazakhstan - Kazakh Honey Cake (Medovik)
Iran - Persian Love Cake
China - Chinese Steamed Sponge Cake (Ma Lai Go)

Australia & Oceania

Samoan -Coconut Cake
Guam - Chamorro Latiya (Layered Custard Cake)
Tuvalu - Tuvaluan Banana Cake

Europe

United Kingdom (UK) - British Victoria Sponge Cake:
Latvia - Riga Honey Spice Cake
Monaco - Riviera Lemon Delight

Caribbean

Guyana - Exotic Spice Fruit Cake
US Virgin Islands - US Virgin Islands Coconut and Rum Cake
Trinidad and Tobago - Trinidadian Black Cake

South America & Latin America

Bolivia - Bolivian Milk Cake (Torta de Leche)
Colombia - Colombian TresLeches Cake
Belize - Belizean Coconut Tart

North America

Montana, USA - Huckleberry Cake
Izamal, Yucatan - Yucatecan Chocolate Cake
Vancouver, Canada - Canadian Maple Cake

Section IV Pies & Cobblers

Africa

Algeria- Algerian Date Pie
Seychelles -Banana Coconut Cobbler
Rwanda- Sweet Potato Pie

Asia

Vietnam - Coffee Pie
Taiwan - Pineapple Cobbler
Hong Kong- Egg Custard Tart

Australia & Oceania
Solomon Islands- Coconut Cream Pie
American Samoa -Banana Cream Pie
Tokelau - Coconut Pie

Europe
Portugal - Pastel de Nata (Custard Tart)
Hungary- Dobos Torte (Layered Sponge Cake)
Finland - Lingonberry Pie

Caribbean
Grenada- Nutmeg Cake
Dominican Republic - Leches Cake
Bahamas- Guava Duff

South America & Latin America
Chile -Chilean Apple Cobbler
Bonaire-Dutch Apple Pie
Costa Rico - Pineapple Cobbler

North America
New Mexico-US Biscochitos
Toronto, Canada - Butter Tart
Chichen Itza (Mexico) - Mexican Flan

Section V Cookies
Africa
Swaziland – Babazekhaya
Ethiopia - DaboKolo Cookies
Tanzania- Kashata Cookies

Asia
Japan - Matcha Green Tea Cookies
Singapore-KuehBangkit Cookies
South Korea-Dasik Cookies

Australia & Oceania
Kiribati - TeKawawong
Tonya - Tonya Coconut
Palau-Banana Bread Cookies

Europe
France - French butter cookies
Croatia- Croatian Kiflice
Belarus -Belarus Almond Nut Cookies

Caribbean
Jamaica - Jamaican Coconut Drops
St. Kitts & Nevis-Guava Thumbprint Cookies
Bermuda - Bermuda Rum Delights

South America & Latin America
Ecuador-Ecuadorian Dulce Delights
Venezuela- Vibrant Venezuelan Crumbles
Panama- Panamanian Coconut Delights

North America,
Colorado- US Mountain Bliss Cookies
Montreal, Canada-Maple Pecan Delights of Montreal
TULUM, Mexico- Coconut Lime Bites

Section VI Ice Cream

Africa
Western Sahara- Sahrawi Tea Ice Cream
Zambia- Pineapple and Ginger Ice Cream
Kenya-Masala Chai Ice Cream

Asia
India- Mango Kulfi
Nepal- Almond and Rose Ice Cream
Indonesia- Durian Ice Cream

Australia & Oceania
Marshall Islands- Coconut Pandanus Ice Cream
Australia-Lamington Ice Cream
Niue- Coconut Lime Surprise Ice Cream

Europe
Turkey- Sahlep Ice Cream
Belarus- Zapekanka Ice Cream
Italy- Tiramisu Gelato

Caribbean
Cayman Islands- Key Lime Pie Ice Cream
Guadeloupe- Banana Flambé Ice Cream
British Virgin Islands- Tropical Fruit Medley Ice Cream

South America & Latin America
French Guiana- Exotic Fruit Sorbet
Guatemala- Horchata Ice Cream
Nicaragua- TresLeches Ice Cream

North America,
Atlanta- Peach Cobbler Ice Cream
Edmonton- Maple Pecan Ice Cream
La Paz, Baja California- Mango Chamoy Ice Cream

Section VII Pudding

Africa
Morocco- Moroccan Orange Blossom Pudding
Egypt-Umm Ali (Egyptian Bread Pudding)
Botswana- Malva Pudding

Asia
Pakistan-Kheer
Malaysia - Bubur Cha Cha
Macau-Serradura

Australia & Oceania
Papua New Guinea- Saksak
Cook Islands -Boysenberry Fool
Pavlova - A Classic New Zealand Dessert:

Europe
United Kingdom- Christmas Pudding
Spain - Tarta de Santiago
Greece- Balkava

Caribbean
Anguilla-Coconut rice pudding
Puerto Rico- Tembleque

South America & Latin America
Suriname-Bojo
Curacao - Curacao pudding
Paraguay- Budín de Pan

North America
Miami, Florida-Coconut Tapioca Pudding
Ottawa, Canada- Butter Tart Pudding.
CAMPECHE Mexico - Arroz con Leche

Next Step

Introduction

Dear Friend,

Celebrating the joy of healthy eating of global cuisine is essential for a sustainable lifestyle.

When was the last time you had a new food experience? Cooked a new healthy meal, dined at different exotic international restaurants, or shopped at a specialty supermarket?

Embracing different textures, types, and touches of food adds to living a full, fit, and fun lifestyle.

It is often said that books you read or don't read reflect your mindset, your bank, and your credit card statement since reflecting your priorities and what you value. Glancing into your shopping basket at the grocery store or farmer's market reflects your waistline, your taste bud, and your food tendencies.

As a fitness professional, nutrition specialist, and food & culture enthusiast, I am constantly observing other people's food habits in grocery stores and restaurants while managing my own. I find myself curiously observing other people's shopping habits in the checkout aisle, much the way friends and family come over to examine what's on my plate and in glass at a cocktail or dinner party. A wiser statement a friend said to me about food choices is "every time I do grocery shopping, I purchase at least one item I have never tried before" This statement inspires me every day.

A glance into your shopping cart will tell me where you spend most of your time shopping and the quality of the food you are buying, whether it is in between the aisle getting lots of cans, frozen meals, and bagged snacks or on the perimeter of the store getting fresh fruits & vegetables, lean cuts of meats or you explored the international aisle add some variety to your healthy meals.

In college is where my love language of international cuisines & curiosities started. I went to school with students from many nations while sticking to a healthy southern meal plan of cafeteria food for track athletes and surviving the tortuous bayou heat. I was starting to desire geera, masala, curry, jerk, and other tantalizing flavors.

I intentionally started seeking out international students making new friends and embracing new cultures. It was my low-budget way of gathering recipes, tasting new cuisines, and sharing stories about the uniqueness of culture from people from around the world. I quickly discovered almost every culture has a
unique way of preparing two things: bread and rice & peas.

I was intentional about making new friends, I think I met and had a friend from almost every nation that was represented on the LSU campus. I can still remember the taste, the stories shared, and many friends as we connected over meals. We didn't have many resources, and we didn't have much time, yet we found a way to tear down walls of isolation and build bridges with each other through food and stories about family and traditions.

This book is a continuation of the food experiences that have profoundly changed and shaped my lifestyle. This collection of recipes gathered is in a 4-part series. Part 1 – Cookbook, part 2- A Soup book, part 3- Salad book, and Part 4 Smoothie book a total of 195 countries that will be released over 12 months period. It is a gift I have been given in college I now give to you.

Have you ever wondered how unpleasant life would be without good food? Food is an essential requirement for growth and tissue repair. It's equally important that you make nutritious food choices.

It has been proposed that breakfast is the most important food for the day. A healthy choice is another factor. Better breakfast options include a mix of protein, healthy fat, and fiber with little or no added sugar. The food eaten upon waking is used to refuel the body after a prolonged night of fasting and sets the pace for the rest of the day.

Each meal in the day is important to attain and sustain a healthy lifestyle. Research shows that people who eat breakfast have lesser consumption of calories throughout the day, are more likely to gain healthier muscle weight, and are less likely to experience morning fatigue and emotional instabilities.

Lunch is another important part of a day's meal. This is because eating in the afternoon replenishes the depleted energy reserves to enable you to regain focus through the activities of the day. It also supplies glucose to the blood for healthy brain function.

Dinner completes the daily food intake that may be inadequate during the day. Dinner must be also nutritious and lean; to help prepare the body that is going resting stage for a good night's sleep and recovery.

A lifestyle of healthy living is a celebration of healthy eating. Food is good its purpose is to fuel the body with energy to do work, work in the gym or the field, work in the office or at home. Food is also used as a connector, whether among friends at school in the cafeteria or colleagues at lunch in the office, or among families at dinner.

This cookbook consists of 147 recipes for desserts recipes

I invite you to explore each continent and all the nations. That exploration journey starts in this cookbook, and leads to the international aisle in the supermarket, on towards your table and table bud. The ultimate hope is that this new healthy food experience would lead to purchasing a ticket to visit a nation, build connections and make new friends along the way. If for some reason you are unable to travel to another country because of time, money, safety, or the borders are chosen because of a health crisis. You still have an opportunity to experience a new food experience, a new way of eating, and a new way of living through the pages of this book. The Re-center Method Natural Diet Holiday & Christmas Desserts.

Celebrating the joy of healthy eating of global cuisine is essential for a sustainable lifestyle.

Joyfully

Hareldau Argyle King

Founder of Being Elevated Lifestyle

SECTION 1

PASTRIES

AFRCIA

Pastries

Koeksisters — South Africa

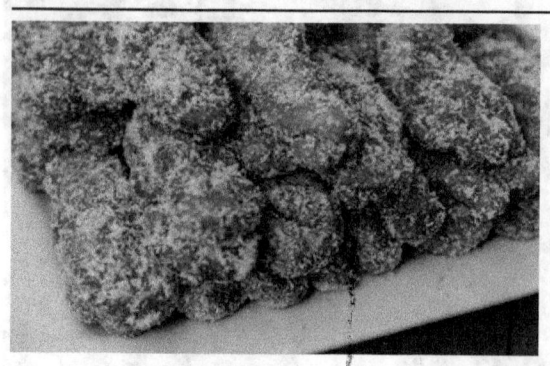

One of the most popular sweet pastry recipes for holiday feasting in South Africa is "Koeksisters." Koeksisters are a traditional Afrikaner treat that are syrup-soaked, twisted pastries with a crunchy exterior and sweet, sticky interior. They are typically enjoyed during special occasions like Christmas and Easter. Here's a recipe for making Koeksisters:

INGREDIENTS

- 4 cups all-purpose flour
- 2 teaspoons baking powder
- 1/4 teaspoon salt
- 2 tablespoons butter, softened
- 1 cup milk
- For the syrup:
- 2 cups sugar
- 1 cup water
- 1/2 teaspoon cream of tartar
- 1 cinnamon stick
- 1 lemon, sliced
- For frying:
- Vegetable oil

DIRECTIONS

1. First if all, Sift the all-purpose flour, baking powder, and salt. Add the softend butter and rub it into the dry ingredients until the mixture resembles fine breadcrumbs.
2. Gradually add the milk, mixing well, until a soft dough forms. Knead until dough becomes soft, elastic and smooth in texture. Cover it with kitchen towel. Let it rest for 1/2 hour at room temperature.
3. While the dough is resting, prepare the syrup. In a saucepan, combine the sugar, water, cream of tartar, cinnamon stick, and lemon slices. Bring the mixture to a boil, stirring until the sugar has dissolved.
4. Simmer for ten minutes. Then cool this syrup completely. Once the dough has rested, roll it out to a thickness of about 5mm (1/4 inch). Cut the dough into strips measuring about 7cm (2.5 inches) long and 1.5cm (1/2 inch) wide. Take each strip and cut a small slit in the center, then twist one end through the slit to form a knot.
5. Heat vegetable oil in a deep pan or fryer to about 180°C (350°F). Carefully lower the koeksisters into the hot oil, frying them in small batches until golden brown and crispy. Remove the koeksisters from the oil using a slotted spoon and drain them on a paper towel.
6. Once all the koeksisters are fried, place them in a shallow dish or tray and pour the cooled syrup over them, making sure they are completely immersed. Allow the koeksisters to soak in the syrup for at least 3 hours or overnight, turning them occasionally to ensure even soaking. Serve the koeksisters at room temperature, either as is or with a sprinkle of desiccated coconut for added flavor and texture. Koeksisters are best enjoyed within a day or two of being made. They are sweet, sticky, and utterly delicious, making them a beloved treat during festive occasions in South

Pastries

Sonhos de banana (banana dreams) – Sao Tome Principle

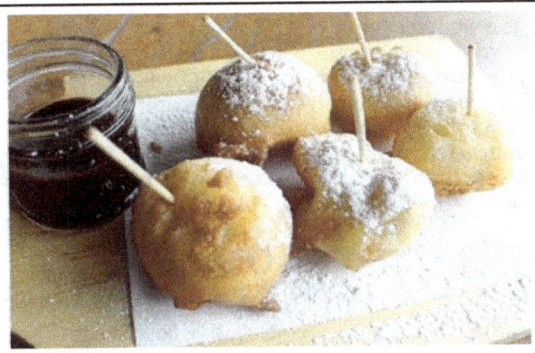

São Tomé and Príncipe is a captivating island nation in Central Africa, known for its breathtaking landscapes and vibrant culture. When it comes to desserts and sweet pastries, this tropical paradise showcases its rich flavors through treats like roças, which are flaky pastries filled with luscious fruit jams, and bolo de mel, a dense and aromatic honey cake.

INGREDIENTS

- 4 ripe bananas, peeled
- Flour 1 cup
- Baking powder 1 teaspoon. ☒ Ground cinnamon 1/2 teaspoon ☒ Salt a pinch.
- Sugar 4 tabspoon
- Milk 1/2 cup
- Oil (for frying
- Sonhos de Banana (Banana Dreams

DIRECTIONS

1. Mash ripe bananas using a fork.
2. In a separate bowl, sift all-purpose flour, baking powder, salt, and cinnamon powder.
3. Add an egg and more cinnamon powder to the mashed bananas, and mix everything well.
4. Gradually pour in some milk until you have a smooth batter.
5. Heat oil in a saucepan or deep fryer
6. 180Ctemprature). Make sure there's enough oil to completely submerge the batter.
7. Use an ice cream scoop or spoon to portion the batter and gently pour it into the hot oil.
8. Fry them in batches so that there is no overcrowding.
9. Fry the banana balls until they turn golden brown, turning them occasionally for even cooking. This usually takes around 3-4 minutes.
10. Use a slotted spoon or tongs to remove the fried banana balls from the oil, and place them on a plate lined with paper towels to absorb excess oil.
11. Fry all balls by repeating this frying process.
12. Once all the banana balls are fried and drained, you can serve them warm. They can be enjoyed as is, or you can dust them with powdered sugar for extra sweetness.
13. Enjoy your freshly made Sonhos de Banana!

Pastries

Chin Chin – Cameroon

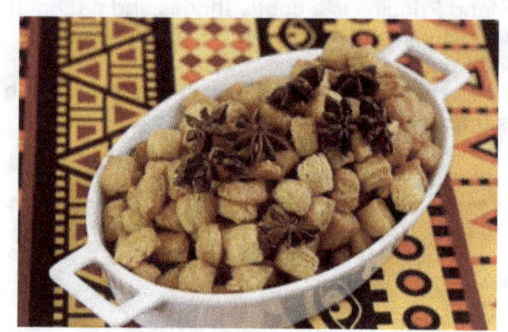

Cameroon is a vibrant country located in Central Africa, known for its rich cultural heritage, diverse cuisine, and warm hospitality. Cameroonian cuisine is a delightful blend of flavors influenced by local ingredients and the country's historical connections with various cultures. While Cameroon is famous for its mouthwatering dishes, it also offers a delectable selection of desserts, including cakes served during special occasions and festive celebrations.

INGREDIENTS

- 2 cups all-purpose flour
- 1/4 cup granulated sugar
- 1/2 teaspoon baking powder
- 1/4 teaspoon salt
- 1/4 teaspoon ground nutmeg
- 1/4 cup unsalted butter, cold and diced
- 1/2 cup milk
- Vegetable oil, for frying

DIRECTIONS

1. In a large mixing bowl, combine the flour, sugar, baking powder, salt, and nutmeg. Mix well.
2. Add the diced butter to the dry ingredients and rub it into the flour mixture with your fingertips until it resembles breadcrumbs.
3. Gradually add the milk, a little at a time, and mix until the dough comes together. Knead the dough lightly for a few minutes until smooth.
4. Roll out the dough on a lightly floured surface to about 1/4 inch thickness. Use a knife or cookie cutter to cut the dough into desired shapes, such as squares or rectangles.
5. Heat vegetable oil in a deep pan or skillet over medium heat. Once the oil is hot, carefully add the cut dough pieces in small batches, frying until golden brown and crispy. Remove with a slotted spoon and drain on paper towels.
6. Allow the Chin Chin to cool completely before serving. It can be stored in an airtight container for several days.
7. Enjoy the delightful crunchiness of Cameroonian Chin Chin as a tasty snack or dessert option!

ASIA

Asian desserts are delightfully diverse and are known for their unique flavors, textures, and presentations. Across the continent, countries have their unique traditional sweets and pastries that play a significant role in holiday feasting and celebrations.

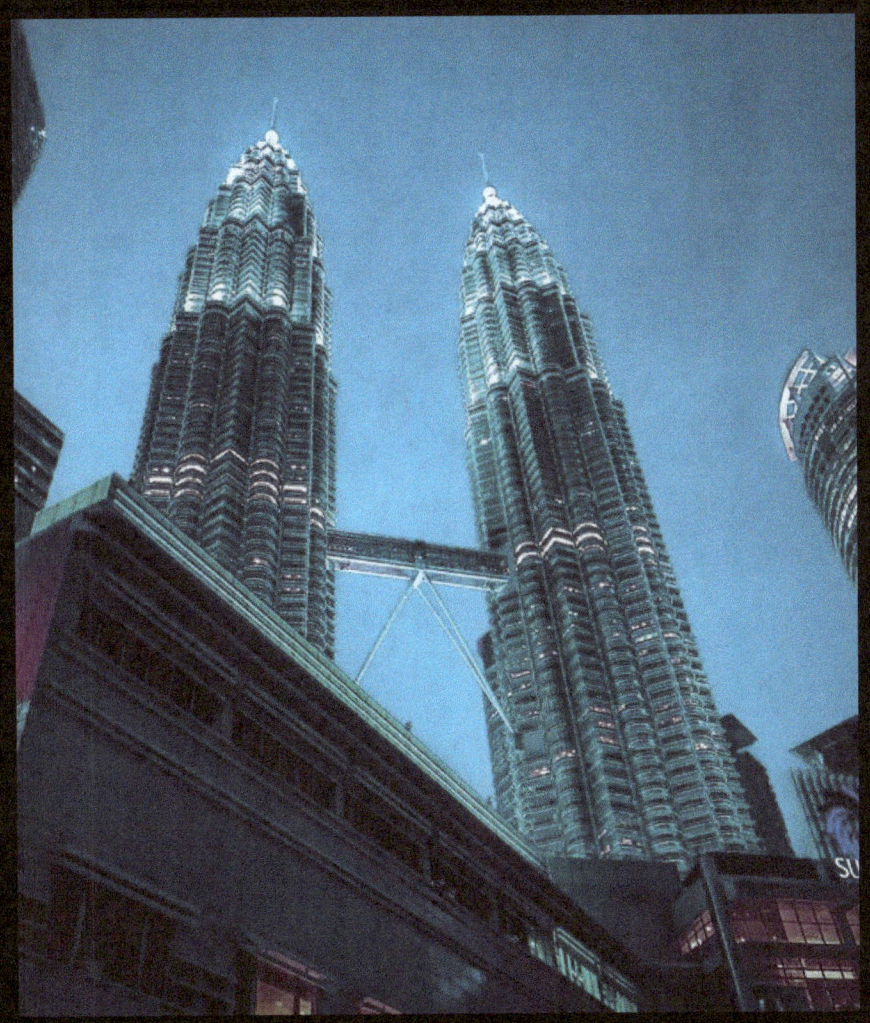

Pastries

Luqaimat – Qatar

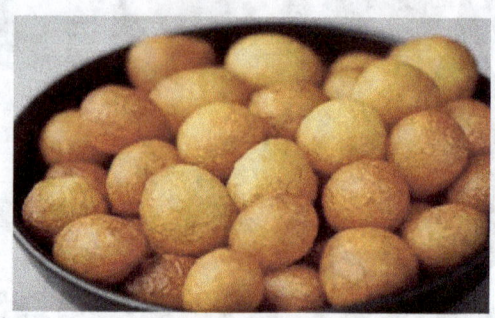

Qatar, a Middle Eastern country, has a rich dessert culture influenced by its Arabian heritage. During festive occasions like Eid al-Fitr, these golden and syrup-soaked morsels are commonly shared among family and friends, symbolizing joy and togetherness.

INGREDIENTS

- All purpose flour 2 cups
- Instant yeast 1 tabspoon
- Corn flour 2 tabspoon ▢ Milk powder 3 tabspoon.
- Salt 1 pinch.
- Sugar 1 tabspoon.
- Lukewarm water 1 cup. ▢ Olive oil 2 tabspoon.
- For sugar syrup
- Water 2 cups
- Sugar 2 cups
- Lemon juice 1 teaspoon ▢ Honey 1/3 cup.

DIRECTIONS

1. Mix flour, instant yeast, salt, milkpowder, cornflour, sugar in a bowl. Pour water gradually and mix until all well combined.
2. Then add oil and knead until a sticky and smooth dough forms. The dough must be sticky. It consistency should be like pancake batter. Neither thick nor thin.
3. Cover it with a plastic wrap. let it rest for one hour.
4. Meanwhile prepare sugar syrup.
5. Add sugar, water in a sauce pan. let it cook until sugar dissolves. Keep flame medium. Add lemon juice and honey.
6. Stir well and set aside for later use.
7. With the help of ice cream scoop drop small balls into hot oil.
8. Fry until golden brown. Keep flame low Flip with a slotted spoon so that they cook evenly from inside.
9. Avoid to over crowd pan for best results.
10. When cooked, discard from oil and place on kitchen towel to absorb excess oil. Then transfer balls into honey syrup
11. Let it rest for 1 hour.

Pastries

Khanom Buang – Thailand

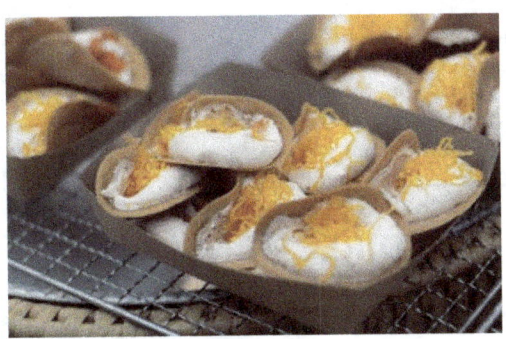

Thailand is famous for its delectable desserts and sweet pastries, Thai sweet pastry is "KhanomBuang," also known as Thai crispy pancakes. This delightful treat consists of crispy shells filled with a sweet and savory mixture of coconut cream and mung bean paste.

INGREDIENTS

- For the crispy shells:
- 1 cup rice flour
- 1 tablespoon all-purpose flour
- 1 1/2 cups coconut milk
- 1/2 cup water
- 1/2 teaspoon salt
- 1/2 teaspoon turmeric powder (for a touch of color, optional)
- Vegetable oil (for frying)

For the filling:

- 1/2 cup mung beans (split, skinless)
- 1 cup coconut cream
- 3/4 cup palm sugar or brown sugar
- 1/4 teaspoon salt
- For the topping (optional):
- Grated coconut, steamed and salted

DIRECTIONS

Crispy Shells:

1. In a mixing bowl, combine rice flour, all-purpose flour, salt, and turmeric powder (if using)
2. Add water and coconut milk to the dry ingredients. Stir continuously until you have a smooth thin consistency batter. Leave it for 15-20 minutes. Filling:
- Rinse the mung beans and soak them in water for about an hour. Drain the water.
- In a saucepan, bring water to a boil and add the soaked mung beans. Cook until the beans are soft and can be easily mashed with a fork.
- Drain any excess water and mash the cooked mung beans.
- In a separate pan, combine coconut cream, palm sugar, and salt. Cook over low heat until the sugar dissolves, and the mixture thickens slightly.
- Add the mashed mung beans to the coconut cream mixture. Stir well and cook for a few more minutes until the filling thickens to a spreadable consistency. Turn off heat. Cool down it at room temperature.

Assembling:

1. Heat a non-stick pan over medium heat. Take a small amount of vegetable oil and ensure it is evenly spread.
- Pour a thin layer of the batter onto the pan, tilting the pan to spread it into a round shape. Cook until the edges become crispy and lift easily from the pan.
- While the shell is still soft and pliable, place a spoonful of the mung bean filling in the center of the pancake.
- Fold the pancake over the filling to form a half-moon shape, and then fold it again to create a quarter-circle. Press gently to seal the edges.
- Remove the filled crispy pancake from the pan and repeat the process with the remaining batter and filling. Optional Topping: Steam the grated coconut and sprinkle a pinch of salt over it.

1. Serve the KhanomBuang warm with the optional coconut topping if desired. Enjoy this delightful Thai sweet pastry with family and friends!

Pastries

Mont Lone Yay Paw (Sweet Floating Rice Balls) - Myanmar

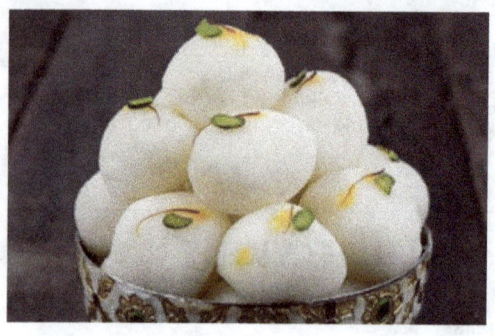

Discover the captivating flavors of Myanmar, a Southeast Asian gem. Its desserts are a taste sensation, transporting your taste buds. Don't miss the chance to experience the sweet side of Myanmar's culinary treasures

INGREDIENTS

For the filling:
- Grated jaggery or (palm sugar)cut into small cubes.1 cup
- For the pastry
- Glutinous Rice flour 2 cups.
  Rice flour 4 tab spoon
  salt 1/2 teaspoon.
  Water 1 -1/2 cup.

DIRECTIONS

1. In a mixing bowl, combine the rice flour and salt in a mixing bowl. Mix well.
2. Add water gradually and knead until you get a smooth and soft dough. if it's too dry then add more water. If too thick then add a little more rice flour.
3. Divide the dough into 25 small parts and make small balls out of it.
- Take a small ball of dough and use a rolling pin to flatten it into a thin circle that is about 5 inches across
4. Place a spoonful of the jaggery or palm sugar onto the center of the dough circle.
5. Fold the sides of the dough over the filling to create a half-moon shape. Press the edges together firmly so that jaggery cubes may seal firmly inside.
6. Repeat the process until you make 25 balls.
7. Boil water in a large-sized sauce pan.
8. Add balls one by one.
- In the beginning, they will sink down to the bottom, but when they're fully developed, they will rise up and float on the water's surface. That's why they got their name
9. Take them out and rinse them with water.
- Garnish with grated coconut and enjoy!
10. By the way, It is enjoyed as a sweet treat or snack, often served with a cup of tea.

Australia and Oceania

Pastries

Firi-Firi – French Polynesia

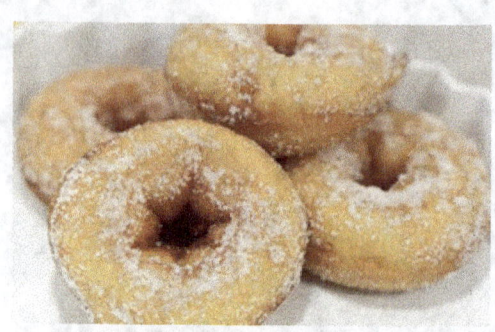

French Polynesia is a captivating tropical paradise in the South Pacific, known for its breathtaking beauty and rich cultural heritage. The region's desserts embody a fusion of French patisserie techniques and Polynesian flavors. FiriFiri, coconut doughnuts with a touch of sweetness, are a popular breakfast or snack choice.

INGREDIENTS

- All purpose flour 2 cups
- Instant yeast 1 tabspoon.
- Caster sugar 2 tabspoon
- Vanilla bean 1/2
- coconut milk 1/4 cup
- coconut water (at 85 F) 1/2 cup
- Oil for frying
- For garnishing icing sugar

DIRECTIONS

1. Pour and dissolve the instant yeast into the coconut water.
2. In the bowl of a stand mixer, Mix all-purpose flour, caster sugar, and vanilla seeds in a bowl.
3. Pour milk flour, sugar, coconut milk, yeast dissolved in the coconut water, vanilla seeds, coconut milk, and yeast with the coconut water addition mixture. Knead until you get a smooth dough.
4. Cover the bowl with a kitchen towel and let it rest for 1 hour or until it doubles in volume.
5. After this dust your working surface with flour.
6. Divide dough into 10 equal parts.
7. Shape them into sausage shape. Fold them so they are shaped like 8.
8. Place parchment paper on a baking sheet.
9. Set these donuts and let them rest for another 1/2 hour.
10. Heat oil in a large saucepan.
11. Deep fry Fri Fri until golden brown from both sides. Place Fri Fri on absorbent paper to drain excess oil
12. Sprinkle icing sugar on top and enjoy!

Pastries

Custard Pie — Fiji

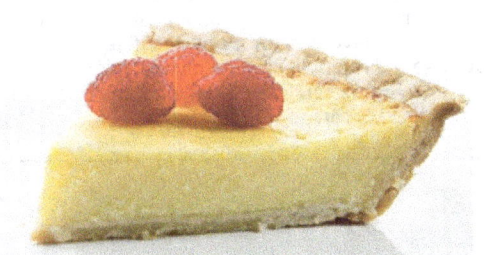

Experience Fiji as you indulge in a diverse array of pastries inspired by the island's rich cultural heritage. Fiji's pastry combines indigenous Fijian, Indian, Chinese, and European influences. Fiji's pastry paradise that will leave you with unforgettable taste sensations and cherished memories.

INGREDIENTS

- 1 1/2 cups all-purpose flour
- Baking powder 2 teaspoon
- Sugar 1/2 cup
- Butter 1/2 cup
- Eggs 2
- vanilla essence 1/2 teaspoon
- Milk 2 cups
- custard powder 2 tabspoon
- sugar 1/2 cup

TOPPINGS

- Sliced fruits of your choice (you can also use cocktail fruits)
- whipped cream 1/2 cup condensed milk 1/4 cup crushed peanuts 2 tabspoon

DIRECTIONS

1. In a mixing bowl, cream together the sugar and butter until creamy. Add the eggs, and vanilla essence and mix until all is well combined.
2. Gradually add the all-purpose flour and knead until you get a smooth dough.
3. Grease a small baking dish, ramekins, or an aluminum tray with oil, butter, or cooking spray. Spread the dough evenly onto the tray, making sure to cover the bottom and sides.
4. Make small holes in the dough using a fork to prevent it from rising during baking.
5. Bake at 180°C (350°F) for 20-25 minutes or until the pastry turns golden brown.
6. While the pastry is baking, prepare the custard filling. In a saucepan, pour 2 cups of milk. In a separate bowl, take some milk and add custard powder, stirring well to avoid lumps.
7. Heat the milk in the saucepan and add sugar, stirring until dissolved. Pour in the custard powder and milk mixture, stirring continuously until the mixture thickens. Let it cool down.
8. Once the pastry is baked, let it cool to room temperature. Pour the prepared custard on top of the pastry.
9. Top the custard with condensed milk, whipped cream, sliced fruits, or crushed peanuts. You can use mangoes as a topping, for example.
10. Refrigerate the pie overnight for best results. Enjoy the delicious Fiji Custard Pie as a delightful dessert that combines a creamy custard filling with a buttery pastry crust and your choice of fruity or nutty toppings

Pastries

Matafaga – Walls and Futuna

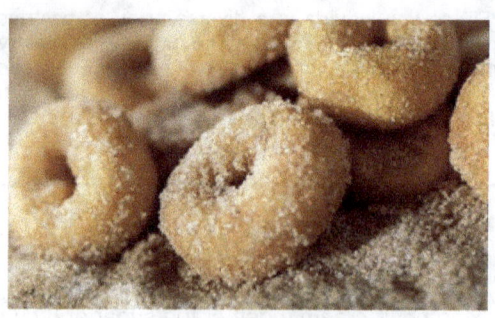

Wallis and Futuna, a French overseas collectivity in the South Pacific, is renowned for its delectable pastries that blend traditional Wallisian flavors with French influences. These pastries showcase the region's cultural diversity and the fusion of Polynesian and French culinary traditions, making them a delight for locals and visitors alike. Matafaga.

INGREDIENTS

- 2 cups all-purpose flour
- 1/4 cup granulated sugar
- 1 teaspoon baking powder
- 1/4 teaspoon salt
- 1/2 teaspoon vanilla extract
- 1/2 cup coconut milk
- 1 large egg
- Vegetable oil, for frying

DIRECTIONS

1. In a large mixing bowl, combine the all-purpose flour, baking powder, salt and sugar and set aside.
2. In a separate bowl, whisk together the coconut milk, egg, and vanilla extract until well combined.
3. Gradually pour the wet ingredients into the dry ingredients while stirring. Mix until a smooth, thick batter is formed.
4. Heat vegetable oil in a deep-fryer or a large, deep pot to 350°F (175°C).
5. With the help of an ice cream scoop, drop a spoonful of the batter into the hot oil carefully. Fry the Matafaga in batches, making sure not to overcrowd the frying pan. Fry the doughnuts for about 2-3 minutes on each side, or until they turn golden brown and are cooked through.
6. Using a slotted spoon, carefully remove the Matafaga from the oil and transfer it to a plate lined with paper towels to allow the excess oil to drain.
7. Optionally, while the Matafaga is still warm, you can roll them in granulated sugar or powdered sugar to add a sweet coating. Serve the Matafaga warm and enjoy these delicious Wallisian deep-fried doughnuts with your family and friends.
8. Note: Matafaga is best served fresh and warm. You can store any leftovers in an airtight container, but they are best consumed on the day they are made.
9. These Matafaga are a delightful treat that showcases the fusion of Wallisian and French culinary traditions, and they are sure to be a hit among locals and visitors alike.

Europe

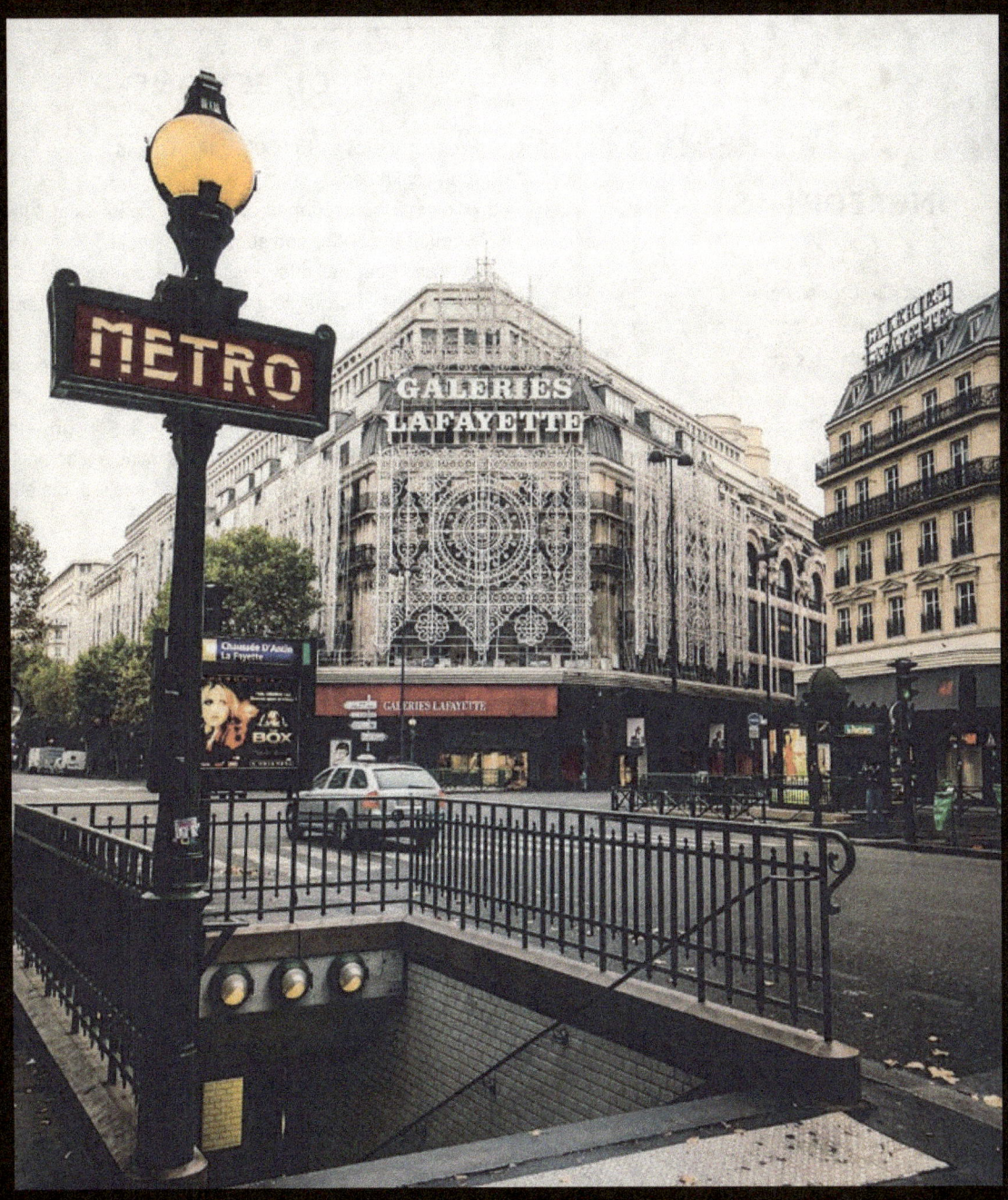

Pastries

Medovik – Ukraine

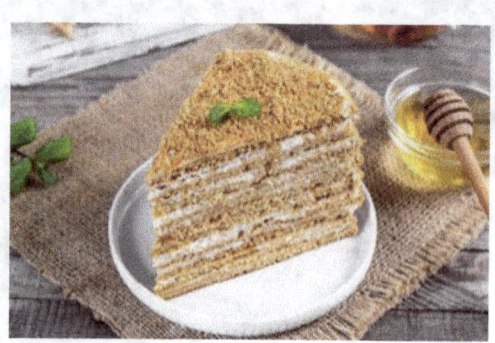

INGREDIENTS

- 4 cups all-purpose flour
- 1 cup unsalted butter, softened
- 1 cup granulated sugar
- 4 large eggs
- 1 teaspoon baking soda
- 1 cup sour cream
- 1 cup sweetened condensed milk
- 1 cup honey 1 teaspoon vanilla extract

Medovik, also known as Honey Cake, is Ukraine's most popular pastry for holiday feasts and celebrations. Ukrainian culinary traditions, symbolizing warmth, hospitality, and the joy of shared moments during festive occasions. Medovik Recipe

Ukraine, a country located in Eastern Europe, boasts a rich culinary heritage and is renowned for its delicious desserts. Ukrainian cuisine is a delightful blend of traditional flavors, unique ingredients, and exquisite pastries.

DIRECTIONS

1. Preheat the oven to 350°F (175°C) and grease and flour a round cake pan.
2. Mix sugar and softened butter until creamy and fluffy cream together the butter and sugar until light and fluffy. Add egg 1 by 1 and beat well after addition of each egg.
3. Mix baking soda in sour cream and add to the batter. Mix again. Add flour and mix with hands until you get a soft and smooth dough. Then divide this dough into eight equal parts.
4. Roll out each portion of dough into a thin circle and transfer it onto the prepared cake pan. Prick the dough with a fork. Bake each layer for about 10-12 minutes or until golden brown. Discard from the oven when cooked immediately to avoid over baking

Cool layers completely.

Syrup preparation.

1. In a saucepan, combine the sweetened condensed milk, honey, and vanilla extract. Cook over low heat, stirring constantly, until the mixture thickens and turns a light caramel color. Turn off heat and let it cool at room temperature.
2. Place one cake layer on a serving plate and spread a generous amount of the honey mixture over it.
3. Repeat this process, layering the cakes with the filling, until all the layers are used, reserving some filling for the top. Spread the remaining honey mixture over the top and sides of the cake, ensuring it is evenly coated. Let the cake sit for a few hours or overnight to allow the flavors to meld and the cake to soften. Serve and enjoy the delicious Ukrainian Medovik! Note: You can also add crushed nuts, such as walnuts or almonds, between the layers for added texture and flavor.

Pastries

Willkommen– Germany

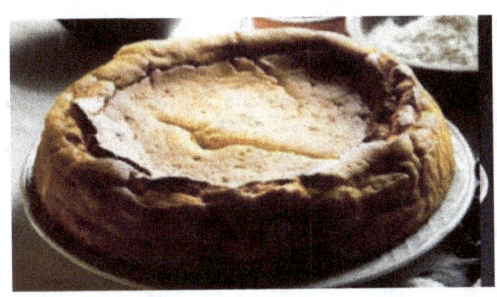

INGREDIENTS

German mouthwatering desserts and pastries are rich in flavors with intricate designs, and time-honored traditions. They are an absolute treat for both the eyes and the taste buds. Dive into the world of German desserts and discover the magic that lies within each delectable bite.

DIRECTIONS

1. Make the dough by combining flour, salt, water, oil, and vinegar in a mixer. Knead until a soft ball forms, let it rest for 60-90 minutes.
2. Heat the oven, soak raisins, peel, core, and slice apples. Place a tablecloth on the work surface to cover it.
3. Roll out the dough thinly on the tablecloth. Spread melted butter, breadcrumbs, apples, raisins, and cinnamon sugar on half of the dough.
4. Fold the dough over the filling to create an envelope shape. Lift and roll the strudel using the tablecloth, ensuring the filling stays inside.
5. Transfer the rolled strudel onto a baking sheet lined with parchment paper. Repeat the process for the second half of the dough and filling.
6. Brush the tops of both strudles with melted butter. Bake until golden brown. It will take a maximum of 30 minutes for its perfect baking.
7. Allow the strudel to cool for 10-15 minutes before slicing. Dust with powdered sugar before serving.

Pastries

Swiss Apple Tart – Switzerland

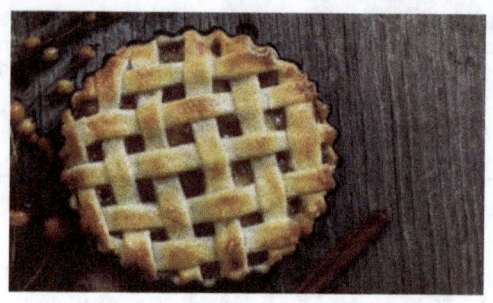

Enjoy warm with a scoop of vanilla ice ream Switzerland, situated in the heart of Europe is known for its breathtaking landscapes, Swiss Alps, and captivating cities, Switzerland is also a haven for all dessert enthusiasts. Switzerland is a pastry paradise where every bite is a sweet symphony of flavors. So, get ready to indulge in the finest Swiss treats that will delight your senses.

INGREDIENTS

- 1 sheet of puff pastry, thawed (store-bought or homemade)
- 2-3 medium-sized apples (such as Granny Smith or Honey crisp), thinly sliced
- 2 tablespoons unsalted butter, melted
- 2 tablespoons granulated sugar
- 1/2 teaspoon ground cinnamon
- Flour, for dusting
- 2-3 tablespoons apricot preserves or jelly

DIRECTIONS

1. Preheat oven to (200°C)
2. Cover the baking sheet with parchment paper.
3. Flatten the puff pastry sheet on a surface lightly dusted with flour
4. Transfer pastry to the prepared baking sheet.
5. Lightly score a border about 1 inch from the edge of the pastry.
6. Arrange thinly sliced apples within the border, overlapping them in a decorative pattern.
7. Mix melted butter, sugar, and cinnamon in a bowl. Brush over the arranged apples.
8. Bake for 20-25 minutes until pastry is golden and apples are tender.
9. Warm apricot preserves or jelly in a saucepan until melted.
10. Remove tart from the oven and brush melted preserves or jelly over the apples.
11. Let it cool before serving.
12. Enjoy warm or at room temperature

CARIBBEAN

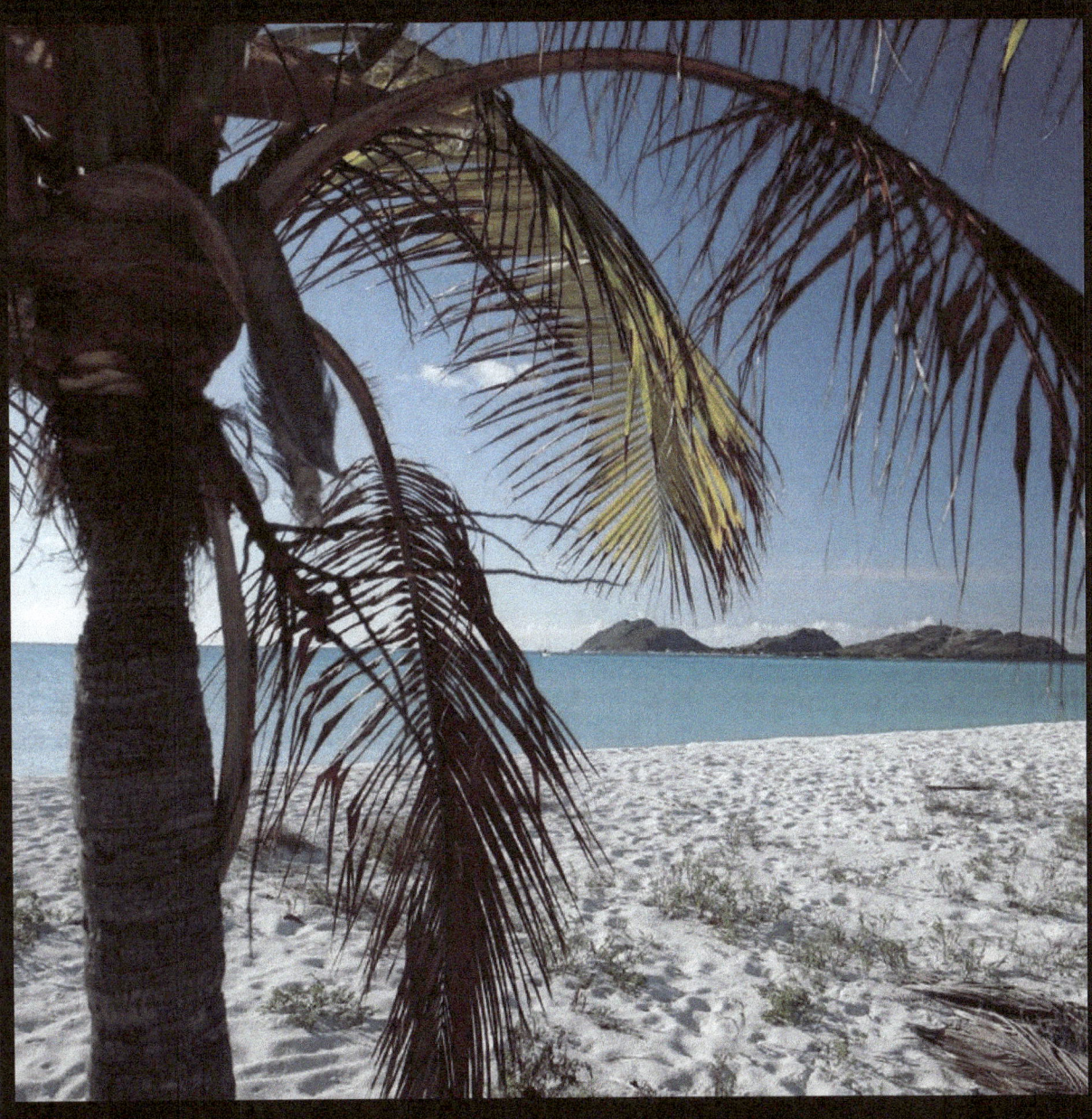

Pastries

Dominica Delight — Dominica

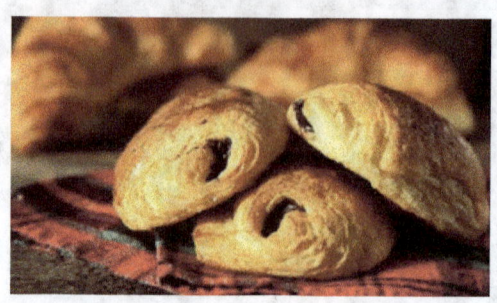

Dominica is renowned for its exquisite desserts, elevating the art of cakes and pastries to new heights. Indulge in this Caribbean island delightful pastries.

INGREDIENTS

- 1 sheet of puff pastry, thawed
- 1/2 cup Nutella (or any chocolate-hazelnut spread)
- 1/4 cup crushed hazelnuts
- 1 tablespoon melted butter
- Powdered sugar (for dusting)

DIRECTIONS

1. Preheat oven to (190°C) for 10-15 minutes.
2. Line a baking sheet with butter paper or parchment paper.
3. Dust flour on the working surface, and unfold the sheet of puff pastry. Using a rolling pin, gently roll out the pastry to smooth out any creases.
4. Spread the Nutella evenly over the entire surface of the puff pastry sheet, leaving a small border around the edges.
5. Sprinkle the crushed hazelnuts over the Nutella, pressing them lightly into the spread.
6. Starting from one end, tightly roll up the puff pastry sheet into a log. Brush the melted butter over the top of the log to add a golden shine.
7. Using a sharp knife, slice the log into 1-inch thick pieces. Place the slices onto the prepared baking sheet, leaving some space between them to allow for expansion.
8. Bake in the preheated oven for about 15-20 minutes, or until the pastries are puffed up and golden brown.
9. Remove the Dominica Delights from the oven and let them cool on a wire rack for a few minutes.
10. Once cooled slightly, dust the pastries with powdered sugar for an extra touch of sweetness.
11. Serve the Dominica Delights warm or at room temperature. Enjoy with coffee or tea
12. These Dominica Delights are sure to impress with their flaky texture, rich chocolate hazelnut filling, and crunchy hazelnut topping. Enjoy!

Pastries

Sweet Pastry — Grenada

Grenada, an island country in the Caribbean, offers a range of delightful desserts that showcase the flavors of the region. Grenadian desserts are a fusion of local ingredients and traditional cooking methods. Enjoy these flavorful delights that represent the unique culinary heritage of Grenada.

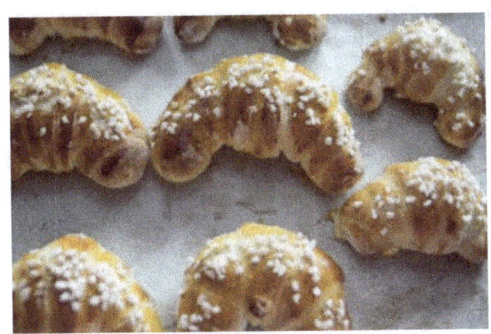

INGREDIENTS

- cups all-purpose flour 2 cups
- salt 1/2 teaspoon
- unsalted butter, chilled and cut into small cubes 1/2 cup
- Granulated sugar 4 tabspoon heaped
- 1 teaspoon vanilla extract
- Cold water, as needed
- Jam or fruit preserves of your choice (e.g., guava, mango, or pineapple)
- Powdered sugar, for dusting (optional)

DIRECTIONS

1. Mix the all-purpose flour and salt in a bowl. Add the chilled butter cubes and use your fingers or a pastry cutter to cut the butter into the flour until the mixture resembles coarse crumbs.
2. Add the granulated sugar and vanilla extract to the flour mixture. Mix well until all well combined.
3. Gradually add cold water, a tablespoon at a time, to the mixture while stirring. Continue adding water and stirring until the dough comes together and forms a smooth ball.
4. Divide the dough into small portions and shape each portion into a ball. Flatten each ball with your hands or a rolling pin to create a round, thin pastry disc.
5. Place a spoonful of jam or fruit preserves in the center of each pastry disc. Fold the disc in half, sealing the edges by pressing them together with your fingers or using a fork to crimp the edges.
6. Preheat your oven to 350°F (175°C). Place the pastry turnovers on a baking sheet lined with parchment paper.
7. Bake the turnovers in the preheated oven for about 15-20 minutes or until they turn golden brown.
8. Once baked, remove the turnovers from the oven and allow them to cool on a wire rack. If desired, dust the turnovers with powdered sugar before serving.

Pastries

Pain Patate — Haiti

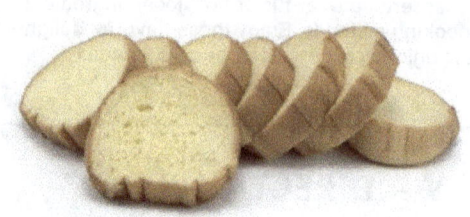

Haiti is a captivating country on the island of Hispaniola. It these desserts reflect Haiti's diverse heritage and the resilience of its people. Each bite tells a story of tradition, creativity, and the joy of savoring life's simple pleasures, inviting you to indulge in the vibrant flavors.

INGREDIENTS

- All purpose flour 1 cup
- mashed sweet potatoes 2 cups
- Brown sugar 1 cup
- Coconut milk 1 cup.
- Butter 1/2 cup
- Vanilla essence 1 and 1/2 teaspoon
- Ground cinnamon 1 teaspoon
- Round nutmeg 1/4 teaspoon
- salt 1/4 teaspoon
- Raisins 1/4 cup

DIRECTIONS

1. Preheat your oven to 350°F (175°C). Grease a baking dish with cooking spray. Place parchment paper on it.
2. In a large mixing bowl, combine the mashed sweet potatoes, brown sugar, melted butter, and vanilla extract.
3. In a separate bowl, whisk together the flour, cinnamon, nutmeg, and salt.
4. Gradually add the dry ingredients to the sweet potato mixture, alternating with the coconut milk.
5. If desired, fold in the raisins to the batter.
6. Pour the batter into the greased baking dish. Spread it evenly with a spatula.
7. Place the dish in the preheated oven and bake for about 45 minutes to 1 hour, or until the top is golden brown and a toothpick inserted into the center comes out clean.
8. After baking, discard the dish from the oven and let it cool at room temperature for a few minutes.
9. Cut the Pain Patate into squares or rectangles and serve warm or at room temperature.
10. Enjoy your homemade Haitian Pain Patate! It's a delicious treat with a unique flavor and texture!
11. South America and Latin America.

South America & Latin America

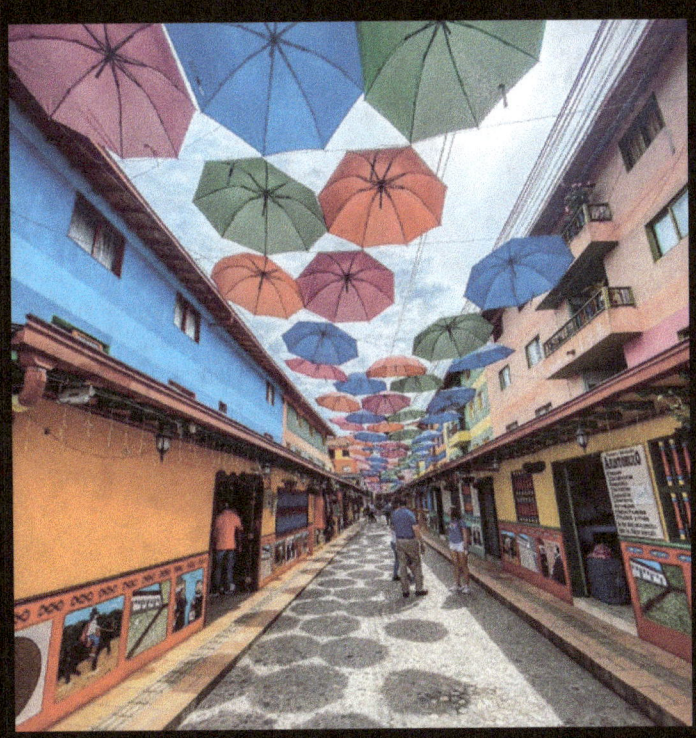

Pastries

Fried Dough — Honduras

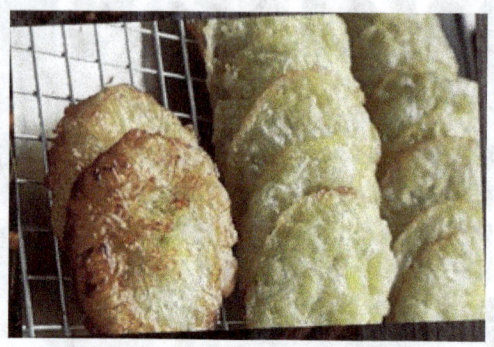

Honduras is a haven for all sweet-toothed adventurers. Immerse yourself inmouthwatering desserts from luscious chocolate truffles to ethereal pastries. Try these delicious central America pastries, where dreams are made of sugar and delightful desserts.

INGREDIENTS

- All purpose flour 2 cups.
- Salt 1/2 teaspoon
- Baking Powder 1/2 teaspoon
- Coconut Oil 2 tabspoon
- Warm Water 1 cup
- Vegetable Oil for frying
- Maple Syrup or honey for Drizzling

DIRECTIONS

1. Sift all-purpose flour, baking powder, and salt. Add coconut oil.
2. Create a well in the center of the dry mixture and pour in water.
3. Gently work the flour and water together to form a dough.
4. Dust your work surface with flour. Knead the dough gently for approximately 5-7 minutes until it becomes soft and flexible.
5. Divide the dough into 12 equal pieces.
6. Grease your hands with a little oil and shape each piece into a uniform ball. Place the balls back in the bowl and cover with a clean cloth. Allow the dough to rest for 45 minutes.
7. Heat oil in a pan over medium-high heat for frying.
8. Dust your work surface with flour. Place dough balls. Flatten each ball with a rolling pin until it becomes approximately 1/8 inch thick and 6 inches in diameter, resembling a tortilla.
9. Using a sharp knife, make 3-4 slits in each tortilla.
10. Fry each tortilla in the heated oil until they turn golden brown on both sides.
11. Once fried, you can drizzle the Honduras fried dough with maple syrup, honey, or maple syrup.

Pastries

Pastel de Nata — Brazil

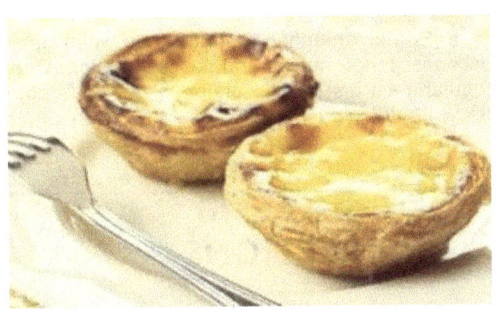

Brazil has a rich culinary heritage and delectable desserts. This pastry is a renowned Portugueseinspired custard tart that has captured the hearts and taste buds of Brazilians far and wide. With its golden, flaky crust delicately hugging a luscious, creamy custard filling, each bite of this pastry transports you to a world of pure indulgence.

INGREDIENTS

- 2 sheets of pre-made puff pastry (or you can make your own) ⊠ Flour (for dusting)
- For the custard filling:
- whole milk 2 cups.
- granulated sugar 4 tabspoon
- 3 tablespoons all-purpose flour 3 tabspoon
- large egg yolks 3
- vanilla essence 1 teaspoon
- Zest of 1 lemon

DIRECTIONS

1. Preheat your oven to 400°F (200°C). Grease a muffin tin or tart mold with butter or cooking spray.
2. Lightly flour a clean surface and roll out the puff pastry sheets until they are slightly thinner. Cut the pastry into squares or circles, depending on the size of your molds.
3. Gently press each pastry square or circle into the molds, making sure to press them into the edges and create a small well in the center.
4. In a saucepan, heat the milk. Keep flame medium. Cook until it simmer lightly.
5. In a separate bowl, whisk together the flour, sugar, and egg yolks until you get a smooth batter.
6. Slowly pour the hot milk into the egg mixture, whisking constantly to prevent the eggs from scrambling.
7. Return the mixture to the saucepan and cook over medium heat, stirring constantly, until it thickens and comes to a gentle boil. Remove from heat and stir in the vanilla extract and lemon zest.
8. Carefully pour the custard filling into the pastry shells, filling them about 3/4 of the way full.
9. Bake in the preheated oven for about 20-25 minutes or until the pastry is golden brown and the custard is set.
10. Remove from the oven and let the Pastel de Nata cool in the molds for a few minutes before transferring them to a wire rack to cool completely.
11. Pastel de Nata is typically enjoyed at room temperature or slightly warm. These custard tarts are wonderfully creamy and have a caramelized top. They are a delightful sweet treat to enjoy with a cup of coffee or tea

Pastries

Alfajores — Argentina

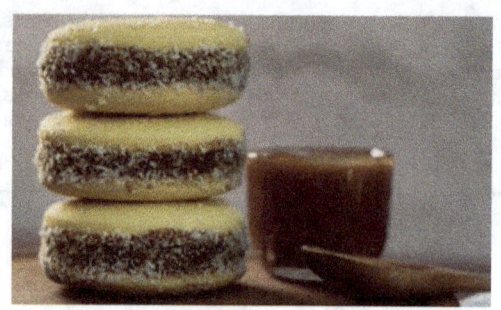

Argentina is a South American country renowned for its diverse landscapes, tango music, and soccer passion. One of the most popular pastries is the Alfajor, a delicious cookie sandwich filled with dulce de leche.

INGREDIENTS

- 200g cornstarch
- 175g all-purpose flour
- 200g unsalted butter
- 150g sugar 3 egg yolks
- 1 tsp vanilla extract
- 1 tsp baking powder
- 1 can of dulce de leche for filling

DIRECTIONS

1. Combine the cornstarch, flour, and baking powder in a bowl.
2. In another bowl, cream the butter and sugar together until light and fluffy.
3. Beat in the egg yolks and vanilla extract.
4. Gradually add the dry ingredients to the wet ingredients, mixing until a soft dough forms.
5. Wrap the dough in plastic wrap and chill for an hour.
6. Roll out the dough and cut out round shapes using a small cookie cutter.
7. Bake at 350F (175C) for about 10-12 minutes.
8. Allow the cookies to cool, then sandwich two cookies together with a generous spoonful of dulce de leche.

North America

North America continent includes the United States, Canada, and Mexico. It is diverse in terms of cultures, landscapes, and cuisines.

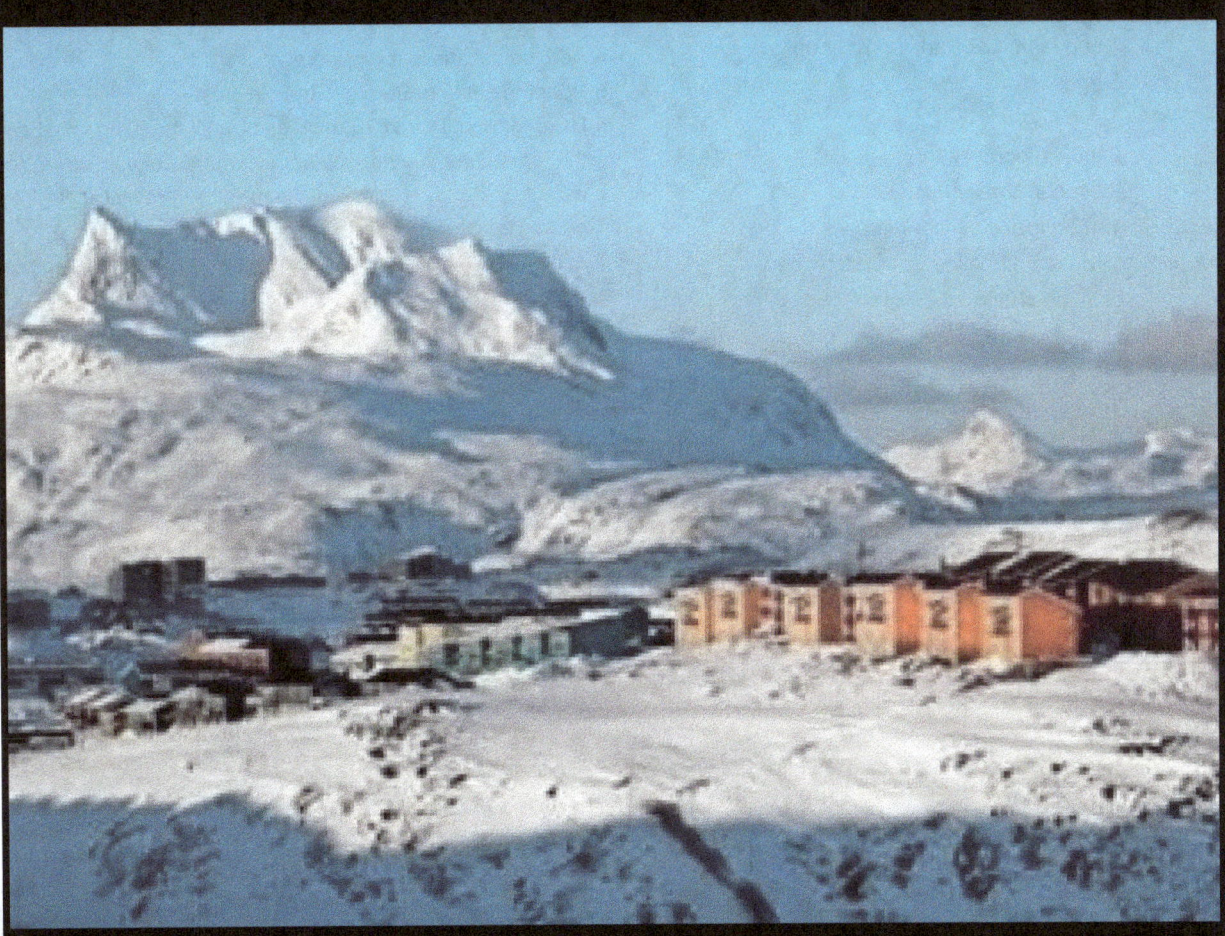

Pastries

Tennessee- Southern Pecan Pie — Nashville

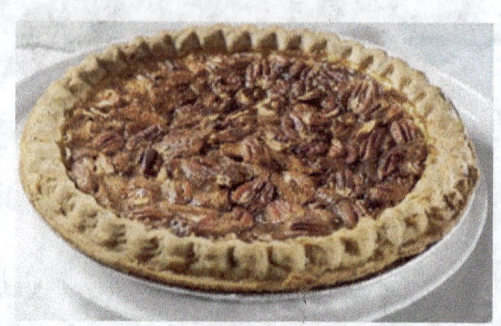

Nashville is the capital city of the U.S. state of Tennessee, known for its vibrant music scene, especially country music. Tennessee is also famous for its Southern cuisine, the Southern Pecan Pie.

INGREDIENTS

- 1 cup Light OR Dark Corn Syrup
- 3 eggs
- 1 cup sugar
- 2 tablespoons butter, melted ◻ 1 teaspoon Vanilla Extract
- 1-1/2 cups (6 ounces) pecans
- 1 (9-inch) unbaked OR frozen deep-dish pie crust

DIRECTIONS

1. Preheat your oven to 350°F (175°C).
2. In a large bowl, beat the eggs lightly while gradually adding the sugar. Continue to beat until the mixture has thickened.
3. Stir in the corn syrup, melted butter, and vanilla extract until well blended.
4. Add the pecans to the mixture.
5. Pour the entire mixture into the pie crust.
6. Bake for about 60 to 70 minutes or until the filling is set and the crust has turned golden brown. You may cover the edges of the crust with aluminum foil to prevent them from getting too brown, if necessary.
7. Allow the pie to cool before serving to ensure the filling sets up nicely.
8. This classic Southern Pecan Pie is a traditional favorite in Tennessee and is sure to satisfy your sweet tooth!

Pastries

Nanaimo Bar — Victoria, Canada

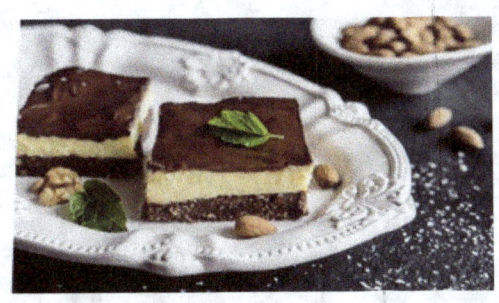

Victoria is the capital city of the Canadian province of British Columbia. It's known for its historic sites, beautiful gardens, and British-influenced culture. A popular dessert in Canada, and indeed in Victoria, is the Nanaimo Bar

INGREDIENTS

- 1/2 cup unsalted butter, melted
- 1/4 cup sugar
- 5 tbsp. cocoa
- 1 egg, beaten
- 1 3/4 cups graham cracker crumbs
- 1 cup coconut
- 1/2 cup finely chopped almonds

DIRECTIONS

1. For the bottom layer, melt the unsalted butter, sugar, and cocoa on top of a double boiler. Add the beaten egg and stir to cook and thicken. Remove from heat.
2. Stir in the graham cracker crumbs, coconut, and almonds. Press firmly into an ungreased 8" x 8" pan.
3. For the middle layer, cream butter, cream, custard powder, and icing sugar together well. Beat until light. Spread over the bottom layer.
4. For the top layer, melt chocolate and unsalted butter over low heat. Once cooled, pour over the second layer and chill in the refrigerator.
5. Remember to always follow safety precautions while cooking or baking. Enjoy making these desserts.

SECTION 11

CUSTARD

AFRICA

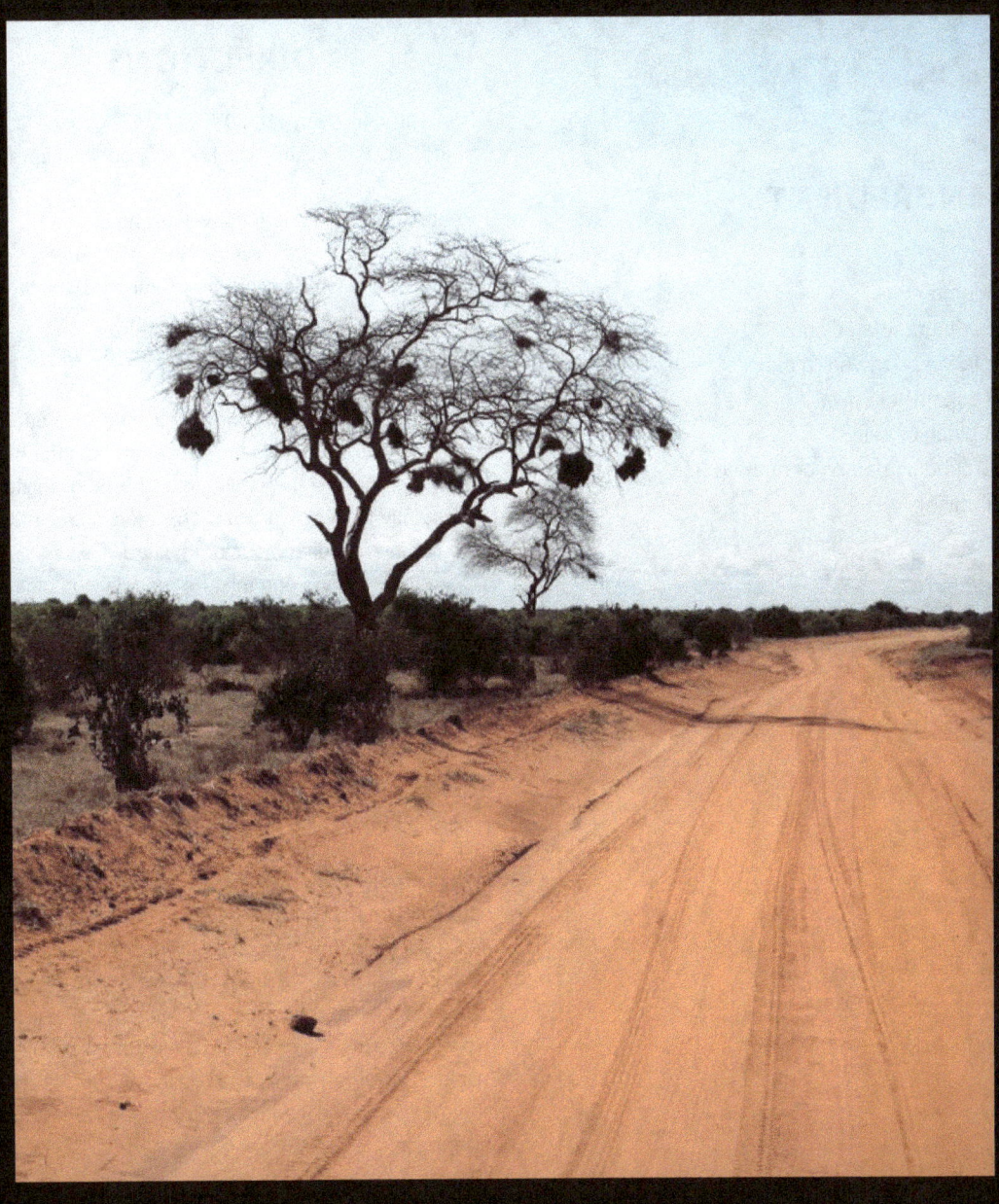

Custard

AsadLeche — Equatorial Guinea

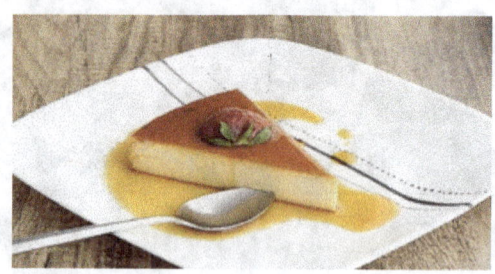

AsadLeche is a delightful African custard, rich in flavor and creamy in texture. This unique dessert is sure to satisfy your sweet tooth and leave you wanting more.

INGREDIENTS

- 6 large eggs
- 1 cup granulated sugar
- 1 tablespoon vanilla extract
- 4 cups whole milk
- A pinch of salt
- Ground cinnamon or nutmeg (for garnish)

DIRECTIONS

1. Preheat your oven to 350°F (175°C). Grease a baking dish or individual ramekins with butter or cooking spray to prevent sticking.
2. Beat eggs well in a large-sized mixing bowl.
3. Gradually add the sugar to the beaten eggs while continuously whisking. Whisk until the mixture becomes smooth and slightly frothy.
4. Add vanilla extract. Do not forget to add salt to enhance the flavor of this custard.
5. Heat the milk in a saucepan over medium heat until it's hot but not boiling. Remove the saucepan from the heat.
6. Slowly pour the hot milk into the egg mixture, stirring constantly to avoid curdling. This step is crucial to achieving a smooth and uniform custard texture.
7. Once the milk and egg mixture are fully combined, strain the custard through a fine-mesh sieve to remove any remaining lumps or egg solids.
8. Pour the strained custard mixture into the prepared baking dish or ramekins.
9. Create a water bath by placing the baking dish or ramekins inside a larger baking pan. Carefully fill the larger pan with hot water, ensuring it reaches about halfway up the sides of the baking dish or ramekins.
10. Gently transfer the water bath to the preheated oven. Bake the custard for approximately 30-35 minutes or until the edges are set, but the center still has a slight jiggle.
11. Remove the custard from the oven and let it cool in the water bath. Once cooled, transfer the custard to the refrigerator to chill for at least a few hours or until fully set.
12. Before serving, sprinkle a dash of ground cinnamon or nutmeg on top of the custard for added flavor and a touch of elegance.
13. Enjoy the luscious AsadLeche custard with friends and family, savoring each creamy spoonful.

Custard

Milk Tart – Ghana

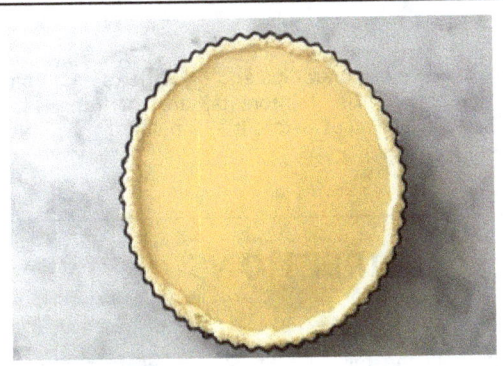

Ghana, a culturally rich African country, is renowned for its diverse and flavorful desserts. Ghanaian desserts showcase a fusion of indigenous flavors and colonial influences. They offer a delightful exploration of the country's culinary heritage, leaving a lasting impression on those who indulge in their delectable flavors.

INGREDIENTS

- 1 liter milk
- 2 cups milk
- 1/2 cup sugar
- 1/2 cup all-purpose flour
- 2 eggs
- 1 teaspoon vanilla extract
- 1 prepared pie crust

DIRECTIONS

1. In a pot, heat the milk until it is just below boiling.
2. In a separate bowl, combine the sugar, flour, and eggs, mixing until smooth.
3. Slowly add a small amount of the warm milk to the egg mixture, stirring constantly.
4. Gradually add the warmed egg mixture to the pot of milk, while stirring continuously.
5. Cook the mixture over low heat until it thickens, ensuring to stir frequently.
6. Remove the pot from heat, stir in the vanilla extract, and let the mixture cool slightly.
7. Pour the milk mixture into the prepared pie crust.
8. Refrigerate the tart before serving.

Custard

Vanilla-Ylang Custard — Comoros

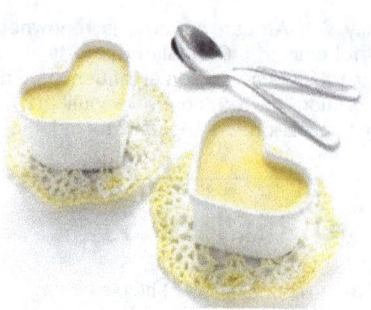

INGREDIENTS

- 2 cups of milk
- 4 egg yolks
- 1/2 cup of sugar
- 1 tsp vanilla extract

The Comoros is a volcanic archipelago off Africa's east coast, known for its coral reefs, rainforests, and perfumeries. In Comoros, the Vanilla-Ylang Custard is a popular.

DIRECTIONS

1. A few drops of ylang-ylang oil.
2. In a pot, heat the milk until it just begins to steam. In a separate bowl, mix the egg yolks, sugar, vanilla, and ylang-ylang oil. Gradually add the warm milk while stirring. Return the mixture to the pot and cook over low heat, stirring until it thickens. Pour into serving dishes and refrigerate before serving.

ASIA

Asian desserts are delightfully diverse and are known for their unique flavors, textures, and presentations. Across the continent, countries have their unique traditional sweets and pastries that play a significant role in holiday feasting and celebrations.

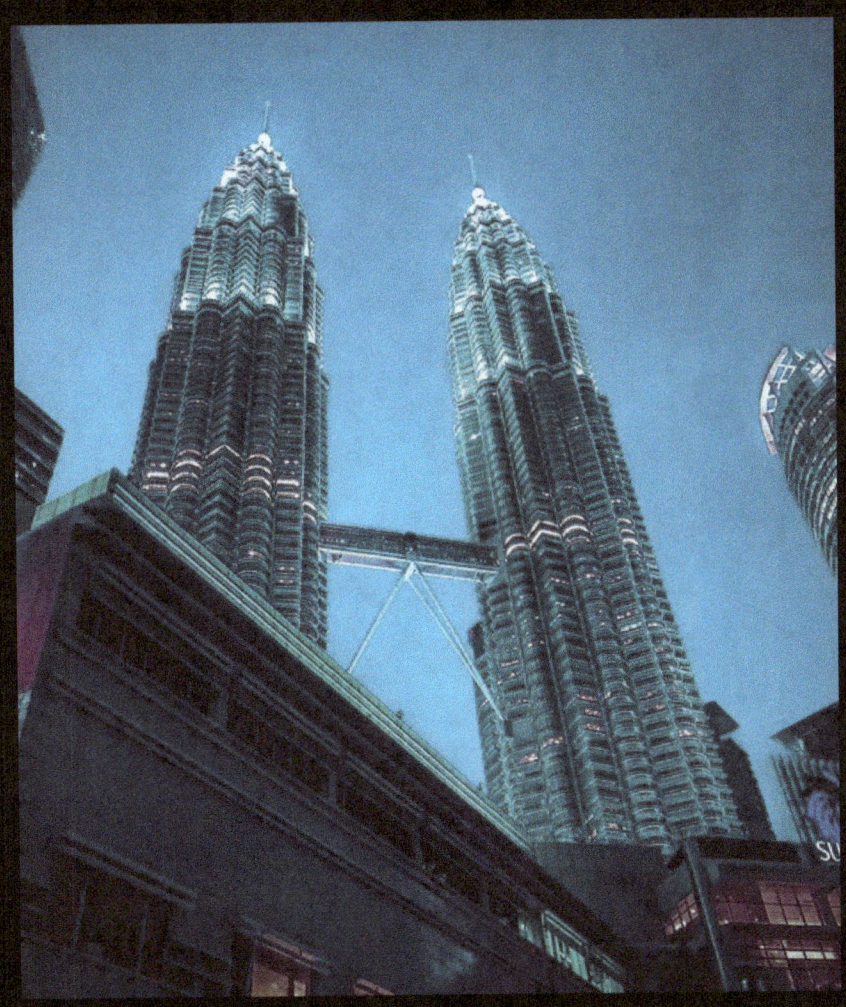

Custard

Malabi — Israel

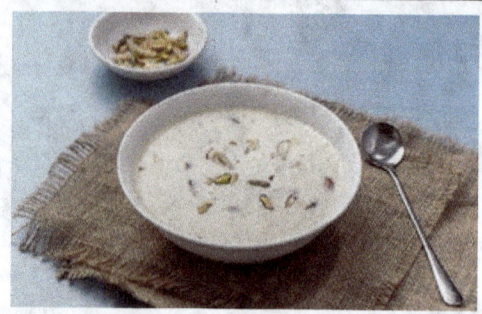

Israel, a small country on the Mediterranean Sea, is rich in history and culture, famous for its biblical sites, archaeological treasures, and delicious food. A classic Israeli custard dessert is Malabi.

INGREDIENTS

- Milk 4 cups, sugar 1 cup
- cornstarch 1/2 cup
- Rose water 1 teaspoon
- Chopped nuts, coconut flakes, and pomegranate seeds for topping

DIRECTIONS

1. Mix a cup of milk with cornstarch until smooth.
2. In a pot, combine the rest of the milk and sugar, bringing it to a boil.
3. Add the cornstarch mixture, and stir continuously until the mixture thickens. Keep the flame low.
4. Remove from heat, add rose water, and pour into serving dishes.
5. Chill until set, then top with nuts, coconut, and pomegranate seeds before serving.

Custard

Boiled Milk Custard Recipe— Mongolia

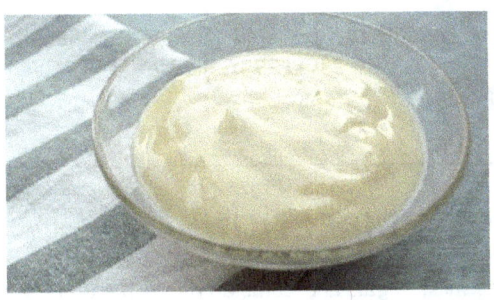

Mongolia is in Central Asia, known for its rugged landscapes, simple life and unique culinary delights. Mongolia also offers a wide variety of desserts that are sure to tantalize your taste buds. They consist of a blend of local ingredients, and ancient recipes.

INGREDIENTS

- 4 cups of milk
- 6 egg yolks
- 3/4 cup of sugar
- 1 tsp vanilla extract
- In a pot, heat the milk until it just begins to steam.

DIRECTIONS

1. In another bowl, mix sugar, egg yolks, and vanilla essence.
2. Gradually add the warm milk while stirring.
3. Return the mixture to the pot and cook over low heat, stirring until it thickens. Pour into serving dishes and refrigerate before serving.

Custard

Gyzgym – Turkmenistan

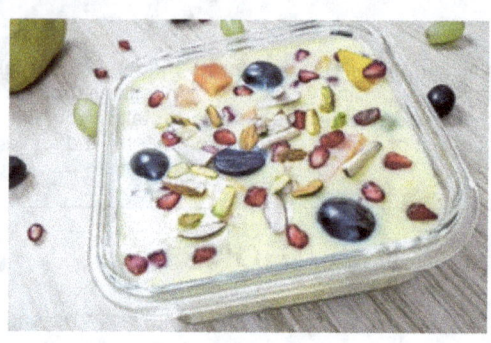

Turkmenistan in Central Asia offers a blend of ancient history, vibrant culture, and a delightful array of desserts with a range of flavors and textures.

INGREDIENTS

- 4 cups of milk
- 1 cup of sugar
- 1/2 cup of cornstarch
- 1 tsp of vanilla extract

DIRECTIONS

1. Combine milk, sugar, and cornstarch in a pot and cook on medium heat, stirring constantly until it thickens.
2. Remove from heat, add the vanilla extract, and pour the mixture into a mold. Let it cool, then refrigerate before serving.

Australia & Oceania

Custard

Coconut Milk Custard — Micronesia

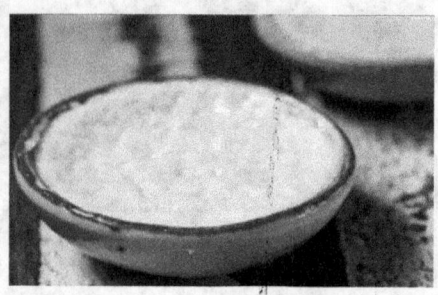

Micronesia is a country in the western Pacific Ocean comprising more than 600 islands known for its beaches, blue lagoons, and extensive coral reefs. A traditional dessert in Micronesia is coconut milk custard.

INGREDIENTS

- 2 cups of coconut milk
- 1/2 cup of sugar
- 4 eggs
- 1 tsp of vanilla extract

DIRECTIONS

1. Preheat the oven to 350°F (175°C). In a bowl, mix together the coconut milk, sugar, eggs, and vanilla.
2. Pour this mixture into a baking dish, place the dish in a water bath, and bake for about 60 minutes, or until set. Let it cool, then refrigerate before serving.

Custard

Coconut Custard Pie — Vanuatu

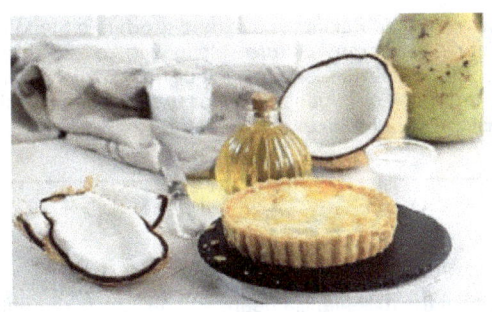

Vanuatu, a South Pacific Ocean nation of a 80 islands. It is known for its stunning beaches and underwater shipwreck sites. One of its popular dessert in is coconut custard pie.

INGREDIENTS

- 1/2 cup flour
- 2 cups milk
- 1 cup shredded coconut
- 3/4 cup sugar
- 2 eggs

DIRECTIONS

1. Preheat the oven to 350°F (175°C). In a bowl, mix together the flour, milk, coconut, sugar, eggs, and vanilla until well combined.
2. Pour this mixture into a pie dish and bake for 45-60 minutes, or until the center is set. Allow to cool before serving.

Custard

Vanilla Flan — New Caledonia

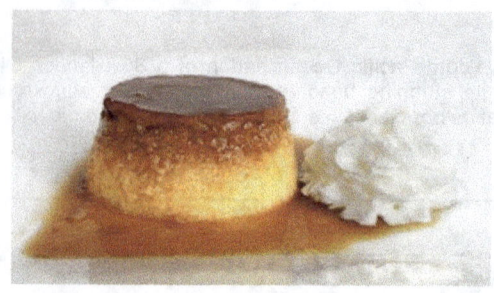

New Caledonia is in the Pacific Ocean, and it offers a blend of natural beauty and vibrant culture, along with a delightful desserts that showcase the island's unique fusion of French, Melanesian, and Pacific influences, savor the essence of this captivating island paradise in every sweet bite.

INGREDIENTS

- 4 cups of milk
- 1 vanilla bean, split and scraped
- 1 cup of sugar
- 6 large eggs
- 1/4 cup of caramel sauce

DIRECTIONS

1. In a pot, heat the milk, vanilla bean, and half the sugar until it just begins to steam.
2. In a separate bowl, whisk together the eggs and remaining sugar.
3. Gradually add the warm milk while stirring. Preheat the oven to 325°F (165°C).
4. In a baking dish, pour the caramel sauce evenly and then pour the mixture over the caramel.
5. Bake for 40- 60 minutes. Let it cool before serving.

Europe

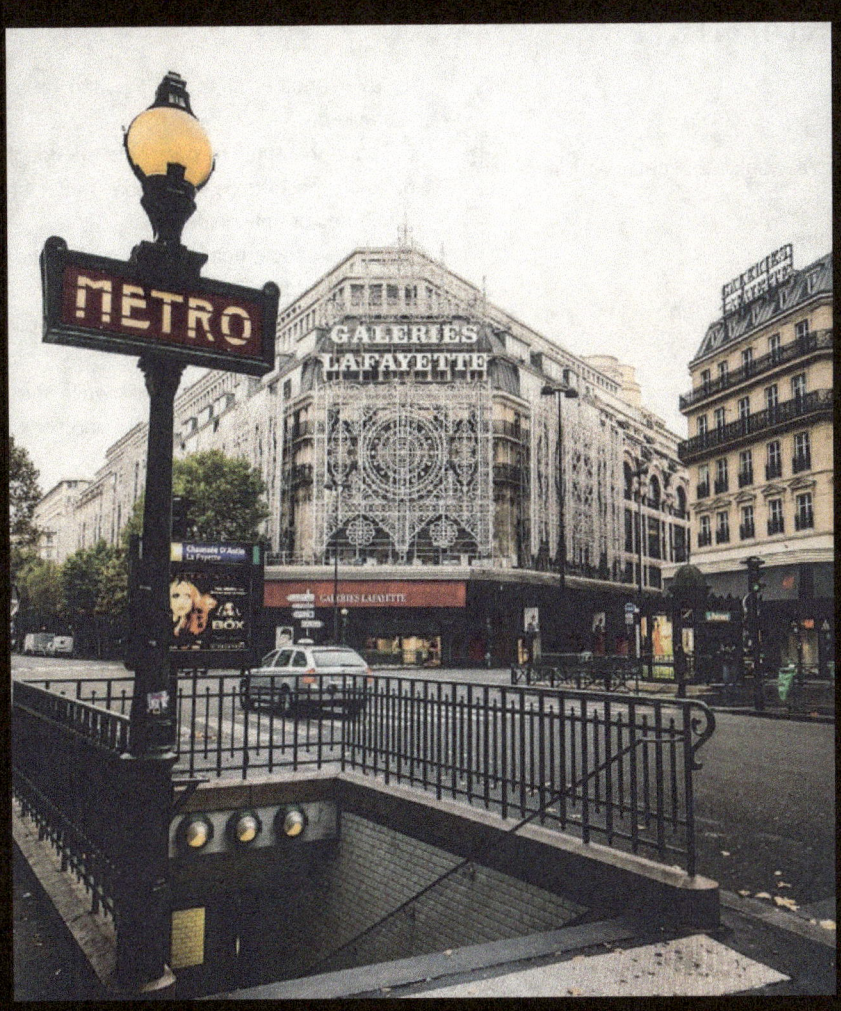

Custard

Viennese Apple Strudel with Vanilla Sauce – Austria

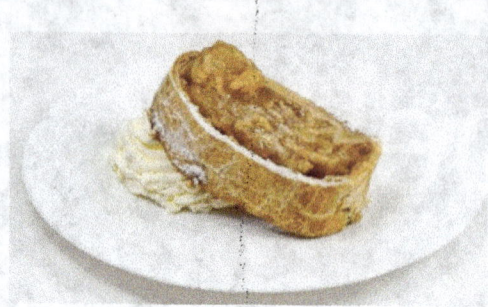

Austria is East Alpine country in the southern part of Central Europe, is famous for its mountain villages, baroque architecture, Imperial history, and rugged alpine terrain. Austria's custard-based dessert is none other than its renowned Viennese Apple Strudel with Vanilla Sauce.

INGREDIENTS

For the strudel:
- Granny Smith apples 2 sliced
- 1/2 cup of sugar
- 1 tsp cinnamon
- 1/2 cup raisins
- 10 sheets of phyllo dough
- 1/2 cup of melted butter

For the vanilla sauce:
- 2 cups of milk
- 1 vanilla bean, split and scraped
- 1/2 cup of sugar
- 4 egg yolks

DIRECTIONS

1. Preheat the oven to 375°F (190°C).
2. In a bowl, combine the apples, sugar, cinnamon, and raisins.
3. Lay out one sheet of phyllo dough and brush it with melted butter.
4. Layer another sheet on top and repeat until all sheets are stacked.
5. Spoon the apple mixture onto the dough and roll it up.
6. Brush the outside with more butter and bake for about 30 minutes or until golden.
7. For the sauce, heat the milk, vanilla bean, and half the sugar until it just begins to steam.
8. In a separate bowl, mix the egg yolks and the remaining sugar.
9. Gradually add the warm milk while stirring.
10. Return the mixture to the pot and cook over low heat, stirring until it thickens.
11. Pour the sauce over the strudel before serving.

Custard

Flan — Spain

Spain, a country on Europe's Iberian Peninsula, is known for its rich culture, beautiful landscapes, and a wide variety of delectable desserts. Flan, a type of custard dessert, is especially popular.

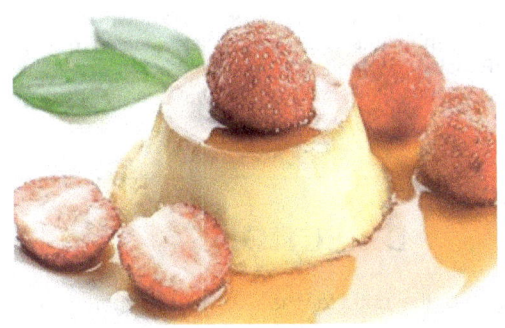

INGREDIENTS

- 1 cup of sugar
- 3 eggs
- 1 can of condensed milk
- 1 can of evaporated milk
- 1 teaspoon of vanilla extract

DIRECTIONS

1. Preheat your oven to 350°F (175°C).
2. In a saucepan, melt the sugar over medium heat until it turns golden, then quickly pour into a round baking dish, swirling to coat the bottom.
3. In a blender, combine the eggs, condensed milk, evaporated milk, and vanilla.
4. Blend until smooth, then pour over the caramelized sugar.
5. Once the oven is preheated, place the dish inside and bake it for 60 minutes.
6. Make sure to cool it down before flipping it onto a plate and serving.

Custard

Tvorojniki— Russia

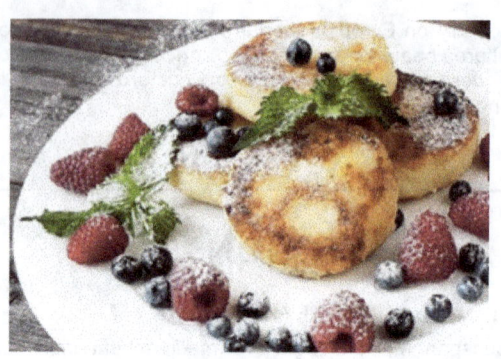

Russia, the largest country in the world, is known for its rich history, iconic landmarks, and traditional Russian desserts. Tvorojniki (Russian Cottage Cheese Pancakes) served with sweetened condensed milk is a favorite.

INGREDIENTS

- 1 lb. (450g) cottage cheese
- 2 eggs
- 3 tablespoons sugar
- 3 tablespoons flour
- 1/2 teaspoon baking powder
- Butter (for frying)
- Condensed milk (for serving)

DIRECTIONS

1. Mix together the cottage cheese, eggs, sugar, flour, and baking powder to form a batter.
2. Heat a pan over medium heat and melt a little butter in it.
3. Scoop the batter into the pan and flatten slightly.
4. Cook until golden brown on both sides.
5. Serve warm, topped with sweetened condensed milk.

CARIBBEAN

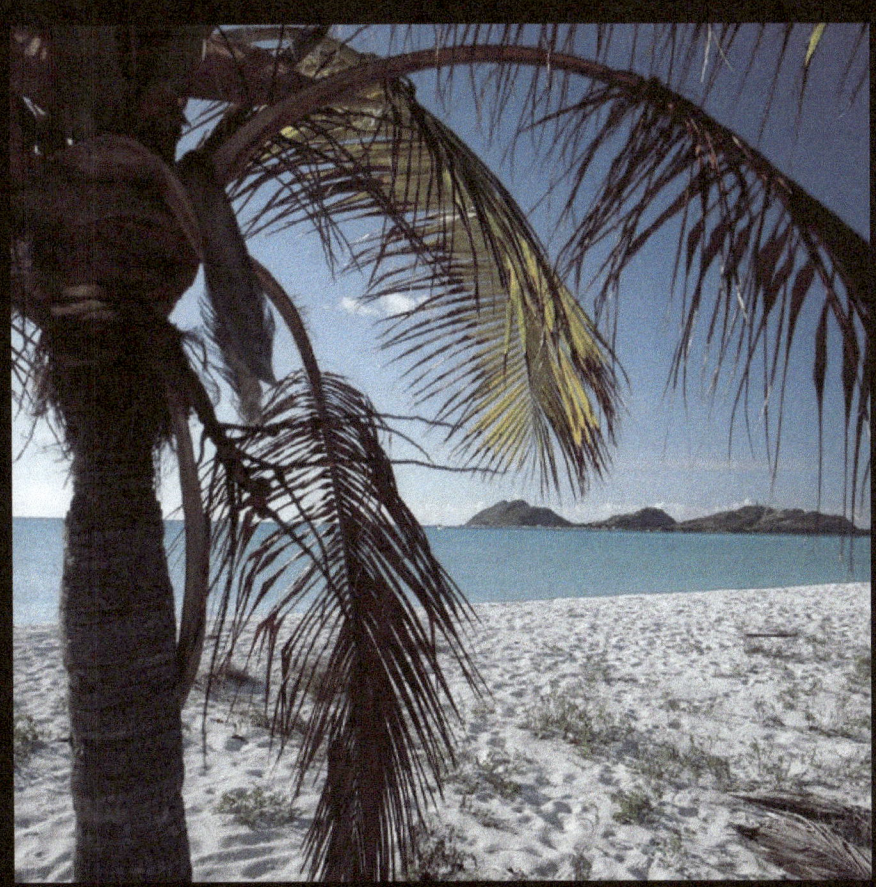

Custard

Bajan Bread Pudding— Barbados

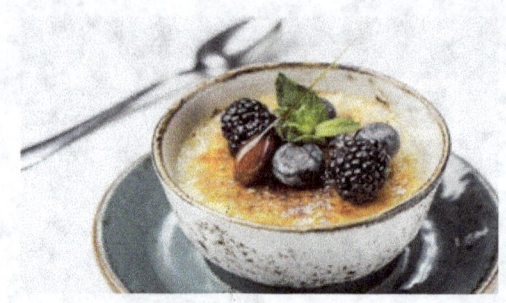

Barbados an eastern Caribbean island, is known for its beautiful beaches, botanical gardens, and the birthplace of rum. A popular custard dessert is Bajan Bread Pudding.

INGREDIENTS

- 5 slices of bread, broken into pieces
- 2 cups of milk
- 2 eggs
- 1/2 cup of sugar
- 1 teaspoon of vanilla extract
- 1/2 teaspoon of nutmeg 1/2 teaspoon of cinnamon
- 1/2 cup of raisins

DIRECTIONS

1. Preheat your oven to 350°F (175°C).
2. In a bowl, combine the bread and milk and let soak for 10 minutes.
3. Stir in the eggs, sugar, vanilla, nutmeg, cinnamon, and raisins.
4. Pour the mixture into a greased baking dish and bake for 45-60 minutes or until set.
5. Serve warm or cold.

Custard

Flan Cubano – Cuba

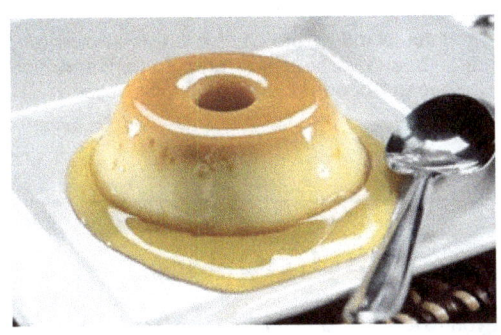

Cuba the largest Caribbean island, is known for its white-sand beaches, rolling mountains, cigars, and saucepan. A popular custard dessert is Flan Cubao.

INGREDIENTS

- 1 cup of sugar
- 6 large eggs
- 1 can of condensed milk
- 1 can of evaporated milk
- 1 teaspoon of vanilla extract

DIRECTIONS

1. Preheat your oven to 350°F (175°C)
2. Melt the sugar over medium heat diverse cuisine until it turns golden
3. In a blender, combine the eggs, condensed milk, evaporated milk, and vanilla blend until smooth, then pour over the caramelized sugar
4. Begin by preheating the oven, then bake the dish for 60 minutes.
5. Once done, let it cool before inverting it onto a plate and serving

Custard

Caribbean Coconut Flan — St Martin

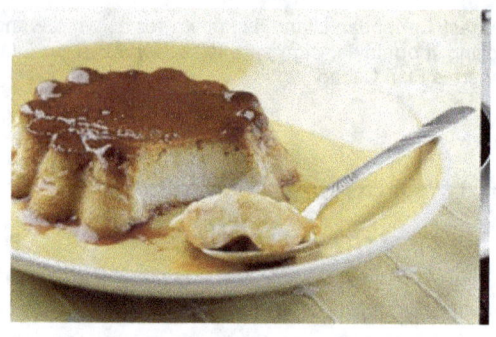

St Martin is a small island in the Caribbean, is known for its vibrant nightlife, beautiful beaches, and French and Dutch influences. Caribbean Coconut Flan is a popular dessert.

INGREDIENTS

- 1 cup of sugar
- 4 large eggs
- 1 can of coconut milk
- 1 can of condensed milk
- 1 teaspoon of vanilla extract

DIRECTIONS

1. Preheat your oven to 350°F (175°C).
2. In a saucepan, melt the sugar over medium heat until it turns golden, then quickly pour into a round baking dish, swirling to coat the bottom.
3. In a blender, combine the eggs, coconut milk, condensed milk, and vanilla.
4. Blend until smooth, then pour over the caramelized sugar.
5. Preheat the oven and bake the dish for 60 minutes.
6. Once baked, allow it to cool before inverting it onto a plate and serving.

South America & Latin America

Custard

Suspiro de Limeña — Peru

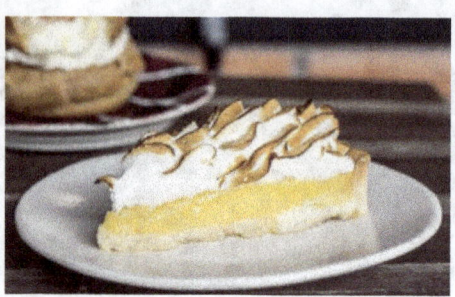

Peru in South America and is known for its rich cultural history, beautiful landscapes, and unique cuisine. A popular dessert here is Suspiro de Limeña (Sigh of a woman from Lima), a sweet custard-like dessert.

INGREDIENTS

- 1 can of condensed milk
- 1 can of evaporated milk
- 4 egg yolks
- 2 cups of sugar
- 1/2 cup of port wine
- 4 egg whites
- Cinnamon powder (for garnishing)

DIRECTIONS

1. In a saucepan, combine the condensed milk, evaporated milk, and egg yolks. Stir continuously until the mixture thickens on medium flame.
2. Pour the mixture into serving glasses and let it cool. In another saucepan, combine the sugar and port wine and cook until a syrup forms.
3. In a separate bowl, beat the egg whites until stiff peaks form, then gradually add the syrup while beating. Spoon this mixture over the cooled custard and garnish with cinnamon.

Custard

Rellenitos de Plátano— Guatemala

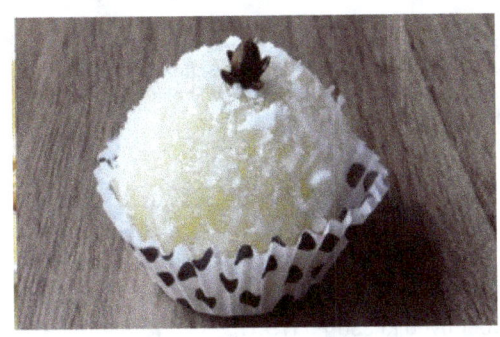

Is a Central America, south of Mexico and is known for its steep volcanoes, vast rainforests, ancient Mayan sites, and vibrant culture. A tasty dessert is Rellenitos de Plátano, a plantain dough filled with sweetened condensed milk.

INGREDIENTS

- 4 ripe plantains
- 1 cup of sweetened condensed milk
- 1/2 teaspoon of cinnamon
- Oil (for frying)
- Sugar (for dusting)

DIRECTIONS

1. Boil the plantains until soft, then drain and mash.
2. Divide the mash into small balls and flatten each ball.
3. Spoon some condensed milk onto each, then fold the plantain dough over the milk to seal it.
4. Heat oil in a pan and fry each ball until golden.
5. Drain on paper towels and dust with sugar before serving.

Custard

Aruban Coconut Pudding– Aurba

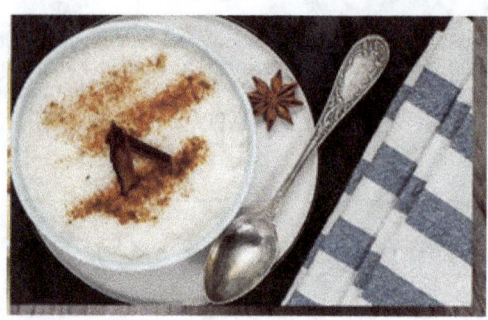

Aruba, a tiny Dutch Caribbean island off the coast of Venezuela, is known for its beauty, dry climate and cactus-strewn landscape. A delicious custard dessert is Aruban Coconut Pudding.

INGREDIENTS

- 1 can of coconut milk
- 1/4 cup of sugar
- 3 eggs
- 1 teaspoon of vanilla extract
- Pinch of salt1/2 cup of shredded coconut

DIRECTIONS

1. Preheat your oven to 350°F (175°C).
2. In a bowl, whisk together the coconut milk, sugar, eggs, vanilla, and salt.
3. Stir in the shredded coconut.
4. Pour into a greased baking dish and bake for 35-40 minutes or until set.
5. Let it cool before serving.

North America

North America continent includes the United States, Canada, and Mexico. It is diverse in terms of cultures, landscapes, and cuisines.

Custard

Akutaq (Eskimo Ice Cream)— Alaska

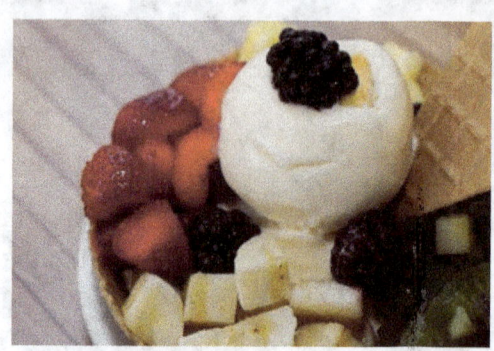

Alaska, the largest state in the U.S., is known for its diverse terrain of open spaces, mountains, and forests, with abundant wildlife and many small towns. It's famous for fishing, hunting, and nature. Akutaq is a popular dessert also known as Eskimo ice cream.

INGREDIENTS

- 1/2 cup of vegetable shortening
- 1/2 cup of sugar
- 1/2 cup of water

DIRECTIONS

1. 1 cup of berries (your choice, but traditionally, salmonberries or blueberries are used)
2. In a bowl, beat the shortening until fluffy.
3. Gradually beat in the sugar and water until well combined.
4. Fold in the berries.
5. Chill in the freezer until solid, then serve.

Custard

Flan — Mexico Zacatecas

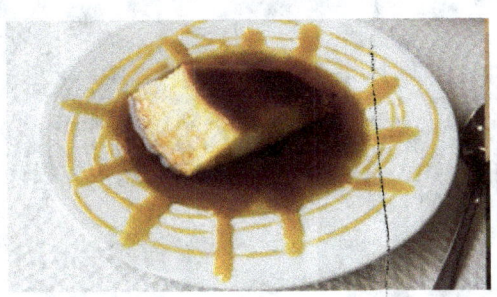

Zacatecanols a city in Mexico, is known for its colonial architecture and vibrant arts scene. Flan Zacatecano, a traditional Mexican custard.

INGREDIENTS

- 1 cup of sugar
- 6 large eggs
- 1 can of condensed milk
- 1 can of evaporated milk
- 1 teaspoon of vanilla extract

DIRECTIONS

1. Preheat your oven to 350°F (175°C).
2. In a saucepan, melt the sugar over medium heat until it turns golden, then quickly pour into a round baking dish, swirling to coat the bottom.
3. In a blender, combine the eggs, condensed milk, evaporated milk, and vanilla.
4. Blend until smooth, then pour over the caramelized sugar.
5. Bake for 60 minutes in the preheated oven.
6. let it cool down to room temperature before flipping it into a serving dish.

SECTION 11
CAKES

AFRICA

Cakes

Nigerian Coconut Cake — Nigeria

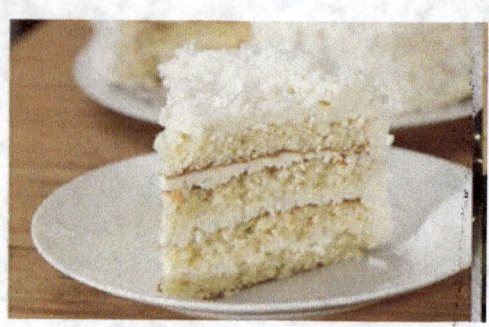

Nigeria is known for its rich and diverse culinary traditions. Nigerian Coconut Cake is a moist and flavorful cake made with coconut milk and grated coconut.

INGREDIENTS

- 2 cups all-purpose flour
- 2 teaspoons baking powder
- 1/4 teaspoon salt
- 1 cup unsalted butter, softened
- 1 1/2 cups granulated sugar
- 4 large eggs
- 1 teaspoon vanilla extract
- 1 cup coconut milk
- 1 cup grated coconut (sweetened or unsweetened, depending on your preference)Recipe:

DIRECTIONS

1. Preheat the oven to (180°C).
2. In a bowl, mix together flour, baking powder, and salt.
3. In a separate bowl, cream butter and sugar. Add eggs one by one. Ensure to mix well after the addition of each egg.
4. Add vanilla extract and coconut milk to the butter mixture, and mix well.
5. Mix dry ingredients to wet ingredients and combine well.
6. Fold in grated coconut.
7. Pour the batter into a greased cake pan. Bake for 40 to 45 minutes at 180C.
8. Let it cool before serving. Enjoy!

Cakes

Togolese Banana Cake — Togo

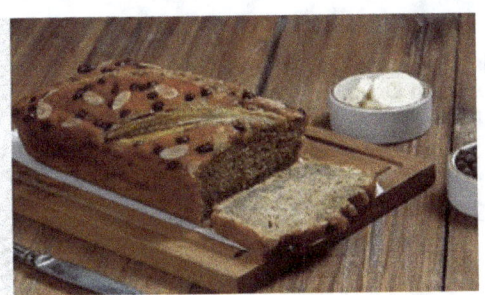

Togo, located in West Africa, has a diverse culinary heritage. Togolese Banana Cake is a delicious and moist cake made with ripe bananas.

DIRECTIONS

1. Preheat the oven to 350°F (175°C).
2. In a bowl, mash ripe bananas with a fork.
3. In a separate bowl, mix flour, baking powder, salt, and cinnamon.
4. Cream butter and sugar in another bowl. Add eggs one at a time, beating well after each addition.
5. Add vanilla extract and mashed bananas to the butter mixture, and mix well.
6. Gently incorporate the dry ingredients into the wet ingredients, adding them gradually and mixing until they are just combined
7. Prepare a greased cake pan and pour the batter into it, then bake for 45-50 minutes or until a toothpick inserted into the center comes out clean
8. Allow it to cool before serving. Enjoy!

INGREDIENTS

- 3 ripe bananas
- 2 cups all-purpose flour
- 1 teaspoon baking powder
- 1/2 teaspoon salt
- 1/2 teaspoon ground cinnamon
- 1/2 cup unsalted butter, softened
- 1 cup granulated sugar
- 2 large eggs
- 1 teaspoon vanilla extract

Cakes

Orange Cake – Morocco

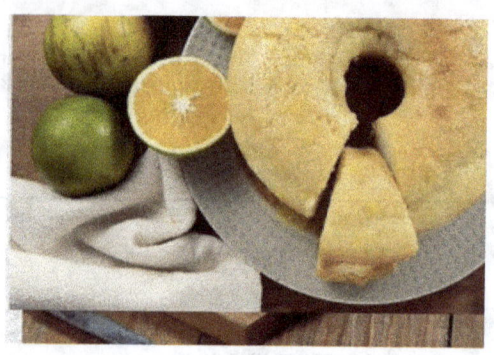

Morocco is renowned for its aromatic spices and unique flavors. Moroccan Orange Cake is a fragrant and moist cake made with fresh oranges and almond flour.

INGREDIENTS

- 2 whole oranges (medium-sized)
- 2 cups almond flour
- 1 cup granulated sugar
- 1 teaspoon baking powder
- 4 large eggs

DIRECTIONS

1. Preheat the oven to 350°F (175°C).
2. In a blender, puree whole oranges.
3. In a bowl, mix almond flour, sugar, and baking powder.
4. Beat eggs in a separate bowl, then add the orange puree and mix well.
5. Combine the wet and dry ingredients gradually, ensuring that they are mixed together just until they are incorporated
6. Grease a cake pan and transfer the batter into it, then bake for 45-50 minutes or until a toothpick inserted into the center comes out clean.
7. Let it cool before serving. Enjoy!

ASIA

Cakes

Persian Love Cake — Iran

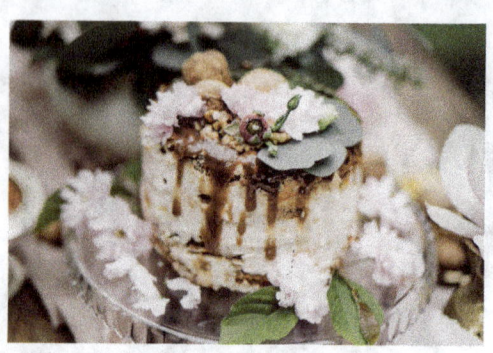

Iran, known for its rich cultural heritage, has a wide variety of traditional desserts. Persian Love Cake is a tasty and indulgent cake with flavors of rosewater, cardamom, and pistachios.

INGREDIENTS

- 1 1/2 cups all-purpose flour
- 1 cup ground almonds
- 1 1/2 teaspoons baking powder
- 1/4 teaspoon salt
- 1 cup unsalted butter, softened
- 1 1/4 cups granulated sugar
- 4 large eggs
- 1 tablespoon rosewater
- 1 teaspoon ground cardamom
- 1 cup plain yogurt
- For decoration:
  - Crushed pistachios
  - Dried rose petals.

DIRECTIONS

1. Preheat the oven to 350°F (175°C).
2. In a bowl, mix together flour, ground almonds, baking powder, and salt.
3. Cream butter and sugar in a separate bowl. Add eggs one at a time, beating well after each addition.
4. Add rosewater, cardamom, and yogurt to the butter mixture, and mix well.
5. Gradually add the dry ingredients to the wet ingredients, mixing until just combined.
6. Pour the batter into a greased cake pan and bake for 40-45 minutes or until a toothpick inserted into the center comes out clean.
7. Let it cool. Decorate with pistachios and rose petals, if desired. Enjoy!

Cakes

Chinese Steamed Sponge Cake (Ma Lai Go) — China

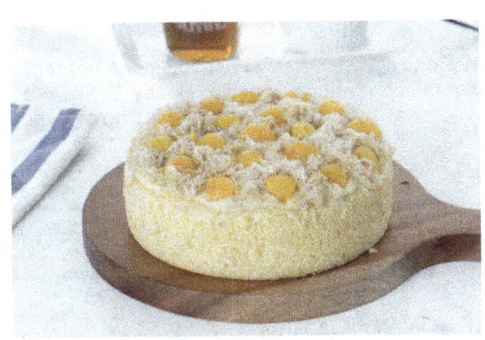

China has a long history of culinary excellence, with a wide range of desserts. Chinese Steamed Sponge Cake, also known as Ma Lai Go, is a fluffy and light cake steamed to perfection.

INGREDIENTS

- 1 cup all-purpose flour
- 1 1/2 teaspoons baking powder
- 1/2 cup granulated sugar
- 3 large eggs
- 1/4 cup mil2 tablespoons vegetable oil

DIRECTIONS

1. In a bowl, mix together flour, baking powder, and sugar.
2. In a separate bowl, whisk eggs, milk, and vegetable oil.
3. Gradually add the dry ingredients to the wet ingredients, mixing until just combined.
4. Pour the batter into greased cake molds.
5. Steam the cakes over high heat for about 20-25 minutes or until a toothpick inserted into the center comes out clean.
6. Let them cool before serving. Enjoy!

Cakes

Kazakh Honey Cake (Medovik) – Kazakhstan

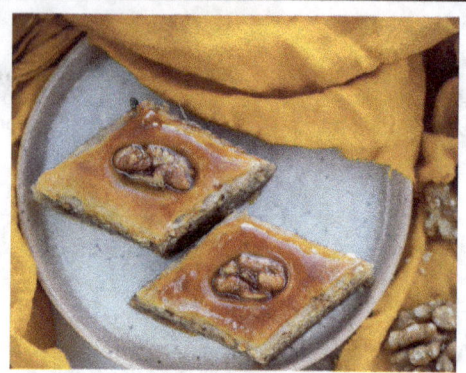

Kazakhstan is in Central Asia, has a rich culinary heritage influenced by its nomadic traditions. Kazakh Honey Cake, also known as Medovik, is a layered cake made with honey and sour cream.

INGREDIENTS

- 2 cups all-purpose flour ⬚ 1 teaspoon baking soda
- 1/4 teaspoon salt
- 1 cup unsalted butter, softened
- 1 cup granulated sugar
- 2 large eggs
- 1/2 cup honey
- 1 cup sour cream ⬚ For the filling:
- 2 cups sweetened condensed milk
- 1 cup unsalted butter, softened

DIRECTIONS

1. Preheat the oven to 350°F (175°C).
2. In a bowl, mix together flour, baking soda, and salt.
3. In a separate bowl, cream butter and sugar. Add eggs one at a time, mixing well after each addition.
4. Add honey and sour cream to the butter mixture, and mix well.
5. Gradually add the dry ingredients to the wet ingredients, mixing until just combined.
6. Divide the dough into several portions and roll each portion into a thin sheet.
7. Bake each sheet for 5-7 minutes until lightly golden.
8. Spread cream or filling of your choice between the layers, and stack them up.
9. Refrigerate the cake for a few hours to allow the layers to soften before serving. Enjoy!

Australia & Oceania

Cakes

Coconut Cake — Samoan

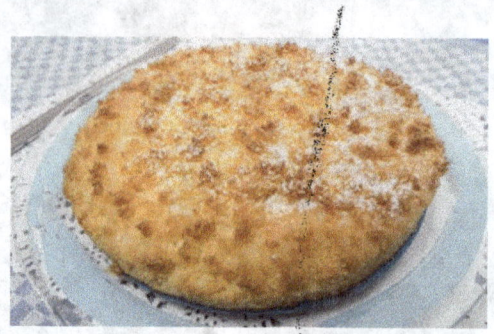

Australia and Oceania have a diverse culinary scene, with influences from indigenous cultures and neighboring countries. Samoan Coconut Cake is a moist and tropical cake made with coconut and pineapple.

INGREDIENTS

- 2 cups all-purpose flour
- 2 teaspoons baking powder
- 1/2 teaspoon salt
- 1/2 cup unsalted butter, softened
- 1 cup granulated sugar
- 2 large eggs
- 1 cup coconut milk
- 1/2 cup pineapple juice
- 1 teaspoon vanilla extract
- 1 cup shredded coconut (sweetened or unsweetened, depending on your preference)
- 1 cup diced pineapple

DIRECTIONS

1. Preheat the oven to 350°F (175°C).
2. In a bowl, mix together flour, baking powder, and salt.
3. In a separate bowl, cream butter and sugar. Add eggs one at a time, mixing well after each addition.
4. Add coconut milk, pineapple juice, and vanilla extract to the butter mixture, and mix well.
5. Gradually add the dry ingredients to the wet ingredients, mixing until just combined.
6. Fold in shredded coconut and diced pineapple.
7. Pour the batter into a greased cake pan and bake for 40-45 minutes or until a toothpick inserted into the center comes out clean.
8. Let it cool before serving. Enjoy!

Cakes

Chamorro Latiya (Layered Custard Cake) – Guam

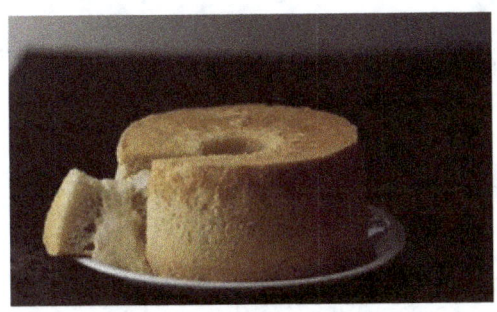

Guam, an island territory in the Pacific, has a unique blend of Chamorro and Spanish influences in its cuisine. Chamorro Latiya is a layered custard cake popular in Guam, made with sponge cake, custard, and cinnamon.

INGREDIENTS

- Sponge cake (prepared or store-bought)
- 4 cups milk
- 1 cup granulated sugar
- 1/2 cup cornstarch
- 1 teaspoon vanilla extract
- Ground cinnamon for dusting.

DIRECTIONS

1. Preheat the oven to 180C.
2. Prepare a sponge cake according to your preferred recipe or using a store-bought mix.
3. Allow the sponge cake to cool completely.
4. Slice the sponge cake horizontally into two or three layers.
5. In a saucepan, prepare a custard mixture using milk, sugar, cornstarch, and vanilla extract. Cook until thickened.
6. Spread a layer of custard on each sponge cake layer and stack them up.
7. Dust the top layer with cinnamon.
8. Refrigerate the cake for a few hours to allow the flavors to meld. Enjoy!

Cakes

Tuvaluan Banana Cake — Tuvalu

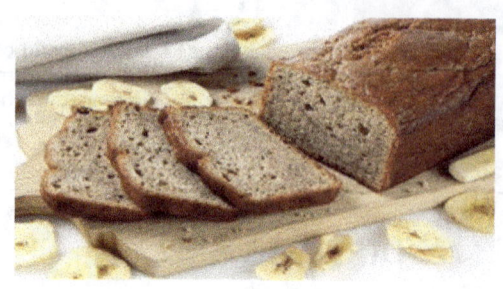

Tuvalu, a small island in the Pacific, has a cuisine influenced by its tropical location. Tuvaluan Banana Cake is a delicious and moist cake made with ripe bananas.

INGREDIENTS

- 3 ripe bananas
- 2 cups all-purpose flour
- 1 teaspoon baking powder
- 1/2 teaspoon salt
- 1/2 teaspoon ground cinnamon
- 1/2 cup unsalted butter, softened
- 1 cup granulated sugar
- 2 large eggs
- 1 teaspoon vanilla extract

DIRECTIONS

1. Preheat the oven to 350°F (175°C).
2. In a bowl, mash ripe bananas with a fork.
3. In a separate bowl, mix flour, baking powder, salt, and cinnamon.
4. Cream butter and sugar in another bowl. Add eggs one at a time, beating well after each addition.
5. Add vanilla extract and mashed bananas to the butter mixture, and mix well.
6. Gradually add the dry ingredients to the wet ingredients, mixing until just combined.
7. Pour the batter into a greased cake pan and bake for 45-50 minutes or until a toothpick inserted into the center comes out clean.
8. Allow it to cool before serving. Enjoy!

EUROPE

Cakes

British Victoria Sponge Cake — United Kingdom (UK)

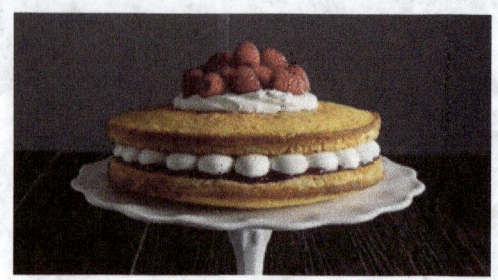

The United Kingdom has a rich culinary tradition, and the Victoria Sponge Cake is a classic British treat. British Victoria Sponge Cake is a light and delicate sponge cake filled with jam and whipped cream.

INGREDIENTS

- 1 cup unsalted butter, softened
- 1 cup granulated sugar
- 4 large eggs
- 2 cups all-purpose flour
- 2 teaspoons baking powder
- 1/4 cup milk
- 1 teaspoon vanilla extract
- Strawberry or raspberry jam for filling
- Whipped cream for filling
- Powdered sugar for dusting

DIRECTIONS

1. Preheat the oven to (180°C).
2. In a bowl, cream together butter and sugar until light and fluffy.
3. Beat eggs, one at a time, into the butter-sugar mixture.
4. Sift flour and baking powder into the bowl and fold gently to combine.
5. Add milk and vanilla extract, and mix until the batter is smooth.
6. Divide the batter evenly between two greased cake pans.
7. Bake for 20-25 minutes or until the cakes are golden and springy to the touch.
8. Allow the cakes to cool completely.
9. Spread jam on one cake layer and whipped cream on top. Sandwich with the second cake layer.
10. Dust with powdered sugar, if desired. Enjoy!

Cakes

Riga Honey Spice Cake – Latvia

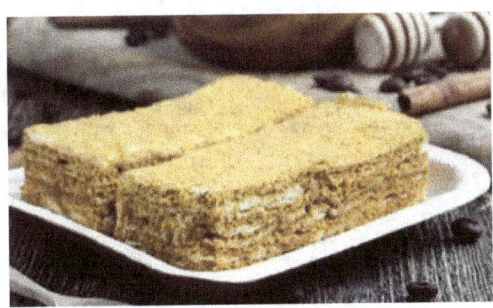

Latvia, located in Northern Europe, has a rich culinary heritage that includes traditional honey-based desserts. Riga Honey Spice Cake, also known as RīgasMēnesītis, is a delightful layered cake made with honey, aromatic spices, and a hint of citrus.

INGREDIENTS

- 1 cup honey
- 1 cup sugar
- 1 cup unsalted butter
- 1 teaspoon ground cinnamon
- 1/2 teaspoon ground ginger ⊠ 1/2 teaspoon ground cloves
- 1/4 teaspoon ground nutmeg
- Zest of 1 orange
- Zest of 1 lemon
- 4 cups all-purpose flour
- 2 teaspoons baking soda
- 1/2 teaspoon salt
- 1 cup sour cream

DIRECTIONS

1. Preheat the oven to 350°F (175°C). Grease and flour a round cake pan.
2. In a saucepan, combine the honey, sugar, butter, cinnamon, ginger, cloves, nutmeg, orange zest, and lemon zest. Heat the mixture over low heat, stirring until the butter has melted and the ingredients are well combined. Remove from heat and let the mixture cool slightly.
3. In a separate bowl, whisk together the flour, baking soda, and salt.
4. Gradually add the dry ingredients to the honey mixture, alternating with the sour cream, beginning and ending with the dry ingredients. Mix well after each addition, until a smooth and thick batter forms.
5. Divide the batter into several portions. Roll out each portion into a thin sheet and transfer them to the prepared cake pan, layering them one on top of the other.
6. Bake for 20-25 minutes or until the layers are lightly golden. Remove from the oven and let them cool completely.
7. In a mixing bowl, whip the sour cream until stiff peaks form.
8. Carefully separate the cooled cake layers and spread a generous amount of whipped sour cream between each layer.
9. Once the layers are stacked, frost the top and sides of the cake with the remaining whipped sour cream. Optionally, you can decorate the cake with honey drizzles or additional spices. Place the cake in the refrigerator for a few hours to allow the flavors to meld and the cake to set.
10. Slice and serve this delectable Riga Honey Spice Cake. Enjoy!

Cakes

Riviera Lemon Delight — Monaco

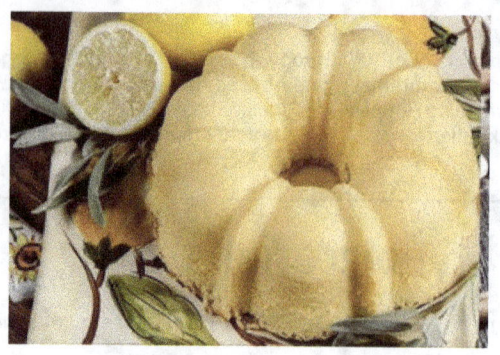

Monaco, a small sovereign city-state on the French Riviera, boasts a cuisine that reflects the vibrant flavors of the Mediterranean. Riviera Lemon Delight is a refreshing and tangy cake that captures the essence of Monaco with its zesty lemon flavor.

INGREDIENTS

- 2 cups all-purpose flour
- 2 teaspoons baking powder
- 1/2 teaspoon salt
- 1 cup unsalted butter, softened
- 1 1/2 cups sugar ⬚ 4 large eggs
- Zest of 2 lemons
- Juice of 2 lemons
- 1 teaspoon vanilla extract
- Powdered sugar, for dusting (optional)
- Lemon slices, for garnish (optional)

DIRECTIONS

1. Preheat the oven to 350°F (175°C). Grease and flour a cake pan.
2. In a bowl, whisk together the flour, baking powder, and salt. Set aside.
3. In a separate bowl, cream the softened butter and sugar until light and fluffy.
4. Add the eggs, one at a time, beating well after each addition.
5. Stir in the lemon zest, lemon juice, and vanilla extract until well combined.
6. Gradually add the dry ingredients to the wet ingredients, mixing until just combined. Be careful not to overmix.
7. Pour the batter into the prepared cake pan and smooth the top.
8. Bake for 40-45 minutes or until a toothpick inserted into the center comes out clean.
9. Remove the cake from the oven and let it cool in the pan for 10 minutes. Then transfer it to a wire rack to cool completely.
10. Once the cake has cooled, dust it with powdered sugar for an elegant touch. You can also garnish with lemon slices if desired.
11. Slice and serve this delightful Riviera Lemon Delight. Enjoy!

CARIBBEAN

Cakes

Tropical Paradise Rum Cake — Caribbean

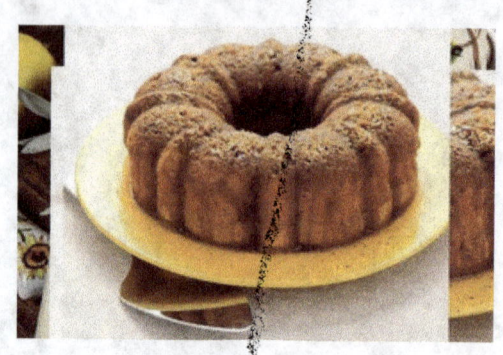

The Caribbean region is renowned for its tropical flavors and the infusion of rum into their delectable desserts.
Tropical Paradise Rum Cake is a luscious and moist cake soaked in rum-infused syrup, offering a taste of the Caribbean.

INGREDIENTS

- 2 cups all-purpose flour
- 2 teaspoons baking powder
- 1/2 teaspoon salt
- 1 cup unsalted butter, softened
- 1 1/2 cups sugar
- 4 large eggs
- 2 teaspoons vanilla extract
- 1/2 cup milk
- 1/2 cup dark rum For the Rum Syrup:
- 1/2 cup unsalted butter
- 1/4 cup water
- 1 cup sugar
- 1/2 cup dark rum

DIRECTIONS

1. Preheat the oven to 325°F (160°C). Grease and flour a Bundt pan.
2. In a bowl, whisk together the flour, baking powder, and salt. Set aside. In a separate bowl, cream the softened butter and sugar until light and fluffy.
3. Add the eggs, one at a time, beating well after each addition.
4. Stir in the vanilla extract, milk, and dark rum until well combined.
5. Gradually add the dry ingredients to the wet ingredients, mixing until just combined. Be careful not to overmix.
6. Pour the batter into the prepared Bundt pan and smooth the top.
7. Bake for 50-60 minutes or until a toothpick inserted into the cake comes out clean.
8. While the cake is baking, prepare the rum syrup. In a saucepan, combine the butter, water, and sugar. Bring to a boil, stirring until the sugar dissolves. Remove from heat and stir in the dark rum.
9. When the cake is done, remove it from the oven and let it cool in the pan for 10 minutes. Then transfer it to a serving plate.
10. While the cake is still warm, use a skewer to poke holes all over the cake. Slowly pour the rum syrup over the cake, allowing it to soak in.
11. Let the cake cool completely before serving, allowing the flavors to meld.
12. Slice and indulge in this Tropical Paradise Rum Cake, transporting yourself to the Caribbean with every bite. Enjoy!

Cakes

Exotic Spice Fruit Cake — Guyana

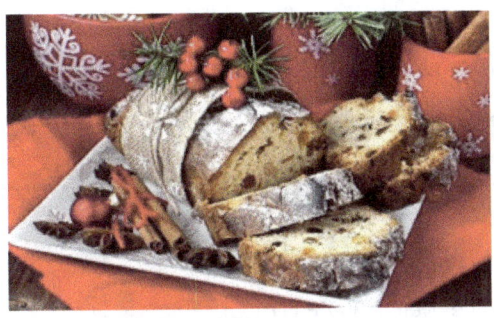

Guyana, boasts a diverse culinary heritage influenced by its multiethnic population. Exotic Spice Fruit Cake from Guyana is a dense and flavorsome fruit cake soaked in a delightful rum infusion.

INGREDIENTS

- 3 cups mixed dried fruits (raisins, currants, cherries, dates)
- 1 cup dark rum
- 2 cups all-purpose flour
- 1 1/2 teaspoons baking powder
- 1/2 teaspoon baking soda
- 1/2 teaspoon salt
- 1/2 teaspoon ground cinnamon
- 1/2 teaspoon ground nutmeg
- 1/2 teaspoon ground cloves
- 1/2 teaspoon ground allspice
- 1 cup unsalted butter, softened
- 1 1/2 cups brown sugar
- 4 large eggs
- 1 teaspoon vanilla extract
- 1/2 cup molasses
- 1/2 cup milk

DIRECTIONS

1. In a large bowl, combine the mixed dried fruits and dark rum. Stir well to ensure all the fruits are coated. Cover the bowl with plastic wrap and let the fruits soak in the rum overnight or for at least 4 hours.
2. Preheat the oven to 325°F (160°C). Grease and line a cake pan with parchment paper.
3. In a separate bowl, whisk together the flour, baking powder, baking soda, salt, cinnamon, nutmeg, cloves, and allspice. Set aside.
4. In a mixing bowl, cream together the softened butter and brown sugar until light and fluffy.
5. Add the eggs, one at a time, beating well after each addition. Stir in the vanilla extract.
6. Gradually add the flour mixture to the butter mixture, alternating with the molasses and milk. Begin and end with the dry ingredients, mixing until just combined.
7. Fold in the soaked dried fruits, along with any remaining rum from the bowl, until well distributed throughout the batter.
8. Pour the batter into the prepared cake pan and smooth the top.
9. Bake for 2-3 hours or until a toothpick inserted into the center comes out clean. If the top of the cake starts to darken too quickly, cover it loosely with aluminum foil.
10. Once the cake is done, remove it from the oven and let it cool in the pan for 15 minutes. Then transfer it to a wire rack to cool completely.
11. For added richness and flavor, you can brush the cooled cake with additional rum.
12. Allow the cake to rest for a day or two before serving. This will allow the flavors to develop and the cake to become moist and flavorful.
13. Slice and savor this Exotic Spice Fruit Cake from Guyana. Enjoy the richness of the fruits and the subtle warmth of the spices with each bite.

Cakes

US Virgin Islands Coconut and Rum Cake — US Virgin Islands

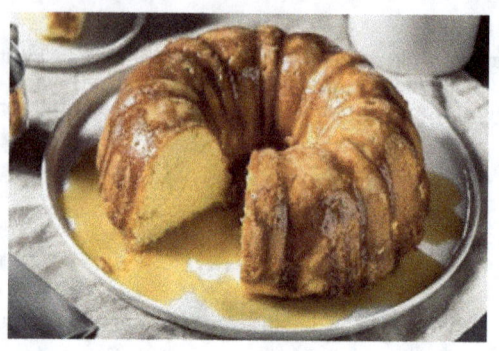

The US Virgin Islands, located in the Caribbean, have a cuisine that combines Caribbean flavors with American influences Virgin Islands Coconut and Rum Cake is a moist and decadent cake infused with coconut and rum.

INGREDIENTS

- 2 cups all-purpose flour
- 2 teaspoons baking powder
- 1/2 teaspoon salt
- 1 cup unsalted butter, softened
- 1 1/2 cups granulated sugar
- 4 large eggs
- 1 cup coconut milk
- 1/2 cup dark rum
- 1 teaspoon vanilla extract
- 1 cup shredded coconut For the rum syrup:
- 1/4 cup dark rum
- 1/2 cup granulated sugar
- 1/4 cup water

DIRECTIONS

1. Preheat the oven to 350°F (175°C).
2. In a bowl, mix together flour, baking powder, and salt.
3. Cream butter and sugar in a separate bowl. Add eggs one at a time, beating well after each addition.
4. Add coconut milk, rum, and vanilla extract to the butter mixture, and mix well.
5. Gradually add the dry ingredients to the wet ingredients, mixing until just combined.
6. Fold in shredded coconut.
7. Pour the batter into a greased and floured cake pan and bake for 45-50 minutes or until a toothpick inserted into the center comes out clean.
8. While the cake is still warm, prepare rum syrup by combining rum, sugar, and water in a saucepan. Bring to a simmer and cook until the sugar is dissolved.
9. Poke holes in the cake using a skewer and pour the rum syrup over the cake, allowing it to soak in.
10. Let the cake cool completely before serving. Enjoy!

Cakes

Trinidadian Black Cake – Trinidad and Tobago

Trinidad and Tobago, located in the Caribbean, has a vibrant culinary culture influenced by African, Indian, and British traditions. Trinidadian Black Cake, also known as Caribbean Christmas Cake, is a rich fruit cake soaked in rum and wine.

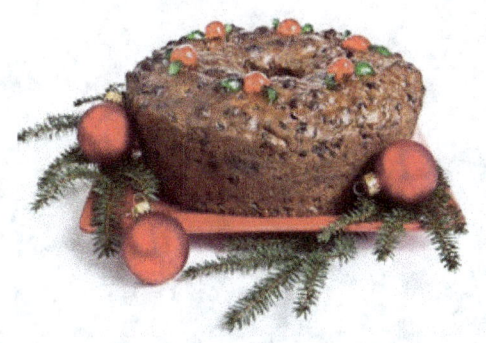

INGREDIENTS

- 3 cups mixed dried fruits (raisins, currants, prunes, cherries, etc.)
- 1 1/2 cups dark rum
- 1 cup unsalted butter, softened
- 1 1/2 cups brown sugar ⊠ 6 large egg
- 3 cups all-purpose flour
- 2 teaspoons baking powder
- 1 teaspoon ground cinnamon ⊠ 1/2 teaspoon ground nutmeg
- 1/2 teaspoon ground allspice
- 1/2 teaspoon ground cloves

DIRECTIONS

1. In a large bowl, mix together soaked mixed fruits (raisins, currants, prunes, cherries) and rum. Let it marinate for at least a week, stirring occasionally.
2. Preheat the oven to 325°F (160°C).
3. In a separate bowl, cream butter and sugar until light and fluffy.
4. Beat eggs, one at a time, into the butter-sugar mixture.
5. Sift flour, baking powder, and spices into the bowl and fold gently to combine.
6. Add soaked fruits, along with any remaining rum, and mix until well distributed.
7. Pour the batter into a greased and lined cake pan.
8. Bake for 2-3 hours or until a toothpick inserted into the center comes out clean.
9. While the cake is still warm, brush it with a mixture of rum and wine.
10. Allow the cake to cool completely before serving. Enjoy!

South America & Latin America

Cakes

Bolivian Milk Cake (Torta de Leche)—Bolivia

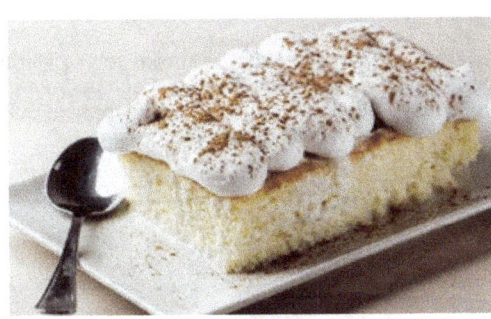

Bolivia, located in South America, has a diverse cuisine that varies by region. Bolivian Milk Cake, also known as Torta de Leche, is a tender and moist cake made with condensed milk.

INGREDIENTS

- 2 cups all-purpose flour
- 2 teaspoons baking powder
- 1/2 teaspoon salt
- 1 cup unsalted butter, softened
- 1 1/2 cups granulated sugar
- 4 large eggs
- 1 can (14 ounces) sweetened condensed milk

DIRECTIONS

1. Preheat the oven to 350°F (175°C).
2. In a bowl, mix together flour, baking powder, and salt.
3. In a separate bowl, cream butter and sugar until light and fluffy.
4. Add eggs one at a time, beating well after each addition.
5. Gradually add the dry ingredients to the butter mixture, alternating with condensed milk, and mix until just combined.
6. Pour the batter into a greased and floured cake pan and bake for 30-35 minutes or until a toothpick inserted into the center comes out clean.
7. Let the cake cool before serving. Enjoy!

Cakes

Colombian TresLeches Cake — Colombia

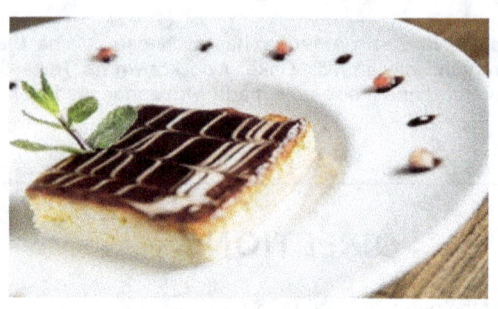

Colombia, located in South America, is known for its vibrant cuisine and diverse desserts. Colombian TresLeches Cake is a sponge cake soaked in a mixture of three types of milk: condensed milk, evaporated milk, and heavy cream.

INGREDIENTS

- 1 cup all-purpose flour
- 1 1/2 teaspoons baking powder
- 1/4 teaspoon salt
- 4 large eggs
- 1 cup granulated sugar
- 1/3 cup whole milk
- 1 teaspoon vanilla extract
- 1 can (14 ounces) sweetened condensed milk
- 1 can (12 ounces) evaporated milk
- 1 cup heavy cream

DIRECTIONS

1. Preheat the oven to 350°F (175°C).
2. In a bowl, mix together flour, baking powder, and salt. In a separate bowl, beat eggs and sugar until light and fluffy.
3. Gradually add the dry ingredients to the egg-sugar mixture, mixing until just combined.
4. Pour the batter into a greased and floured cake pan and bake for 25-30 minutes or until a toothpick inserted into the center comes out clean.
5. In a separate bowl, mix together condensed milk, evaporated milk, and heavy cream.
6. Poke holes in the cake using a skewer and pour the milk mixture over the cake, allowing it to soak in.
7. Refrigerate the cake for a few hours or overnight to allow the flavors to meld. Enjoy!

Cakes

Belizean Coconut Tart — Belize

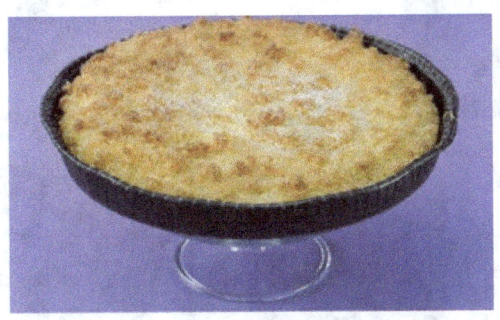

Belize, located in Central America, has a cuisine that combines elements of Caribbean, Mayan, and Mexican flavors. Belizean Coconut Tart is a sweet and creamy tart made with coconut and condensed milk.

INGREDIENTS

- 1 1/2 cups all-purpose flour
- 1/3 cup granulated sugar
- 1/4 teaspoon salt
- 1/2 cup cold unsalted butter, cubed
- 1 can (14 ounces) coconut milk
- 1 can (14 ounces) sweetened condensed milk
- 2 large eggs
- 1 teaspoon vanilla extract

DIRECTIONS

1. Preheat the oven to 350°F (175°C).
2. In a bowl, mix together flour, sugar, and salt.
3. Cut in cold butter until the mixture resembles coarse crumbs.
4. Press the mixture into a greased tart pan, covering the bottom and sides.
5. Bake the tart crust for 10-12 minutes or until lightly golden.
6. In a separate bowl, mix together coconut milk, condensed milk, eggs, and vanilla extract.
7. Pour the filling into the pre-baked tart crust.
8. Bake for an additional 25-30 minutes or until the filling is set.
9. Allow the tart to cool before serving. Enjoy!

NORTH AMERICA

Cakes

Huckleberry Cake — Montana, USA

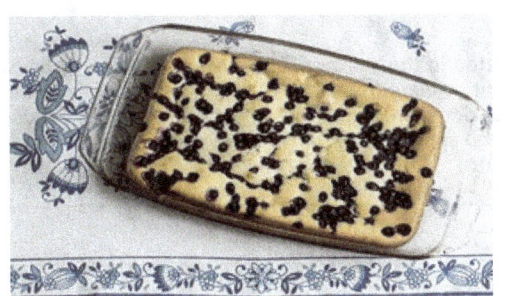

Montana, is known for its picturesque landscapes and hearty cuisine. Huckleberry Cake is a delightful cake made with locally foraged huckleberries.

INGREDIENTS

- 2 cups all-purpose flour
- 2 teaspoons baking powder
- 1/2 teaspoon salt
- 1/2 cup unsalted butter, softened
- 1 cup granulated sugar
- 2 large eggs
- 1 teaspoon vanilla extract
- 1 cup milk 1
- 1/2 cups fresh huckleberries (or frozen, thawed)

DIRECTIONS

1. Preheat the oven to 350°F (175°C).
2. In a bowl, mix together flour, baking powder, and salt.
3. In a separate bowl, cream butter and sugar until light and fluffy.
4. Beat in eggs, one at a time, followed by vanilla extract.
5. Gradually add the dry ingredients to the butter mixture, alternating with milk, and mix until just combined.
6. Gently fold in huckleberries.
7. Pour the batter into a greased and floured cake pan and bake for 40-45 minutes or until a toothpick inserted into the center comes out clean.
8. Let the cake cool before serving. Enjoy!

Cakes

Yucatecan Chocolate Cake — Izamal, Yucatan

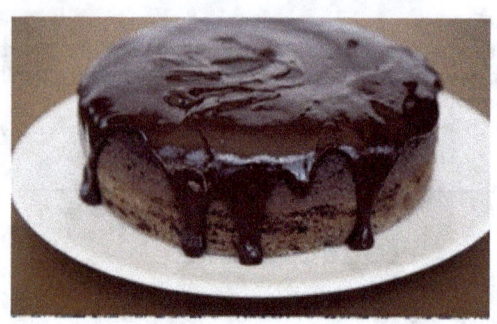

Izamal, located in the Yucatan Peninsula of Mexico, is known for its vibrant culinary traditions. Yucatecan Chocolate Cake is a rich and decadent cake made with traditional Mexican chocolate and spices.

INGREDIENTS

- 1 3/4 cups all-purpose flour
- 3/4 cup unsweetened cocoa powder
- 2 teaspoons baking powder
- 1 1/2 teaspoons ground cinnamon
- 1/4 teaspoon salt
- 1 cup unsalted butter, softened
- 1 1/2 cups granulated sugar
- 4 large eggs 1 teaspoon vanilla extract
- 1 cup milk

DIRECTIONS

1. Preheat the oven to 350°F (175°C).
2. In a bowl, mix together flour, cocoa powder, baking powder, cinnamon, and salt.
3. In a separate bowl, cream butter and sugar until light and fluffy.
4. Beat in eggs, one at a time, followed by vanilla extract.
5. Gradually add the dry ingredients to the butter mixture, alternating with milk, and mix until just combined.
6. Pour the batter into a greased and floured cake pan and bake for 35-40 minutes or until a toothpick inserted into the center comes out clean.
7. Allow the cake to cool completely.
8. Dust with powdered sugar or top with a chocolate ganache, if desired. Enjoy!

Cakes

Canadian Maple Cake — Vancouver, Canada

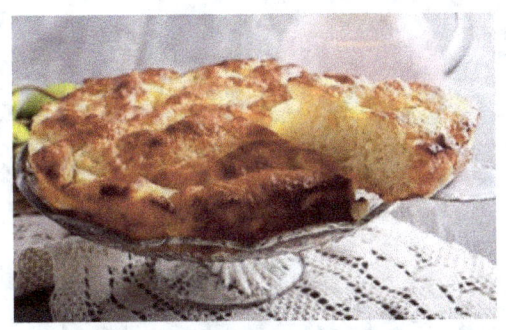

Vancouver, located in Canada, is known for its diverse culinary scene and love for maple syrup. Canadian Maple Cake is a moist and flavorful cake made with real maple syrup.

INGREDIENTS

- 2 cups all-purpose flour
- 2 teaspoons baking powder
- 1/2 teaspoon salt
- 1 cup unsalted butter, softened
- 1 cup granulated sugar
- 4 large eggs
- 1 teaspoon vanilla extract ⌧ 1 cup milk
- 1/2 cup pure maple syrup

DIRECTIONS

1. Preheat your oven to 350°F (175°C). Grease and flour a 9-inch (23 cm) round cake pan or two 8-inch (20 cm) round cake pans to prevent sticking.
2. In a medium bowl, sift the all-purpose flour, baking powder, and salt. Set aside.
3. In a large mixing bowl, cream together the softened unsalted butter and granulated sugar until the mixture becomes light and fluffy.
4. Add eggs and mix well after addition of each egg. Add vanilla extract and mix again.
5. Add dry ingredients to the wet ingredients gradually. Do not add whole milk, add gradually
6. Start by adding about one-third of the dry ingredients, mix until just combined, then pour in half of the milk. Repeat until all the dry ingredients and milk are added, but be careful not to overmix the batter; stop mixing as soon as it becomes smooth and uniform.
7. Gently fold in the pure maple syrup into the batter. The maple syrup will infuse the cake with its unique flavor and contribute to its delightful moistness.
8. Pour the cake batter into the prepared cake pan(s), spreading it evenly with a spatula.
9. Bake the cake in the preheated oven for approximately 25-30 minutes for two 8-inch pans or 35-40 minutes for one 9-inch pan. To check if it's done, insert a toothpick into the center of the cake; it should come out clean with no wet batter sticking to it.
10. Once the cake is baked, remove it from the oven and allow it to cool in the pan(s) for about 10 minutes.
11. Cool cakes on wire rack.
12. Spread the frosting on the cake and decorate as desired. Enjoy the moist and flavorful cake with a delicious maple twist!

SECTION IV

PIES & COBBLERS

AFRICA

PIES & COBBLERS

Algerian Date Pie — Algeria

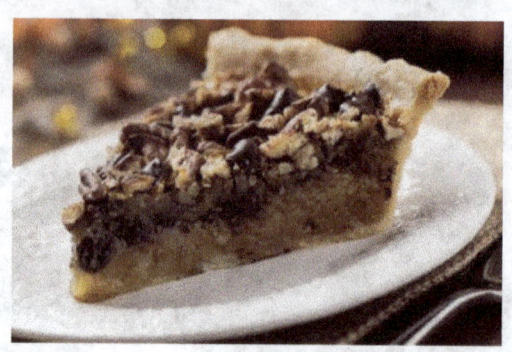

Known for its rich and diverse culinary traditions, Algeria offers a delightful range of desserts. From the famous almond-filled Ka'ak el-Warka pastry to the sweet and flaky Baklava, Algerian desserts showcase the country's love for indulgent treats.

INGREDIENTS

- 2 cups pitted dates, chopped
- 1 cup water
- 1 tablespoon lemon juice
- 1 tablespoon orange blossom water (optional)
- 1 teaspoon ground cinnamon
- 1/2 teaspoon ground nutmeg
- 1/4 teaspoon ground cloves
- 1/4 teaspoon salt
- 1 tablespoon butter
- 1 pre-made pie crust

DIRECTIONS

1. In a saucepan, combine the dates, water, lemon juice, orange blossom water (if using), cinnamon, nutmeg, cloves, and salt.
2. Bring the mixture to a simmer over medium heat and cook for about 10 minutes, or until the dates are softened and the mixture thickens.
3. Remove from heat and stir in the butter until melted. Preheat your oven to 375°F (190°C).
4. Roll out the pre-made pie crust and line a pie dish with it.
5. Pour the date mixture into the pie crust, spreading it evenly.
6. Roll out another piece of pie crust and cut it into strips or shapes to create a lattice or decorative topping.
7. Place the crust strips or shapes over the date filling.
8. Bake in the preheated oven for about 25-30 minutes, or until the crust is golden brown.
9. Remove from the oven and let the pie cool before serving. Enjoy this sweet and spiced Algerian date pie!

PIES & COBBLERS

Banana Coconut Cobbler — Seychelles

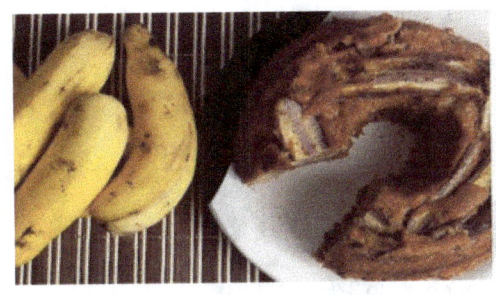

The Seychelles islands are a paradise for dessert lovers. Traditional Seychellois desserts feature tropical flavors such as coconut, pineapple, and banana. Popular treats include Ladob, a creamy coconut dessert, and Tec-Tec, a sweet pastry filled with coconut and sugar.

INGREDIENTS

- 4 ripe bananas, sliced
- 1 cup shredded coconut
- 1/2 cup all-purpose flour
- 1/2 cup granulated sugar
- 1/4 teaspoon salt
- 1/4 cup unsalted butter, melted
- 1/2 teaspoon vanilla extract

DIRECTIONS

1. Preheat your oven to 375°F (190°C).
2. In a bowl, combine the sliced bananas and shredded coconut.
3. In a separate bowl, whisk together the flour, sugar, and salt.
4. Add the melted butter and vanilla extract to the flour mixture, and stir until it forms a crumbly texture.
5. Place the banana and coconut mixture in a baking dish.
6. Sprinkle the flour mixture evenly over the top of the bananas and coconut.
7. Bake in the preheated oven for about 25-30 minutes, or until the topping is golden brown and crispy.
8. Remove from the oven and let the cobbler cool slightly before serving. Serve warm and enjoy the tropical flavors of this Seychellois banana coconut cobbler!

PIES & COBBLERS

Sweet Potato Pie —Rwanda

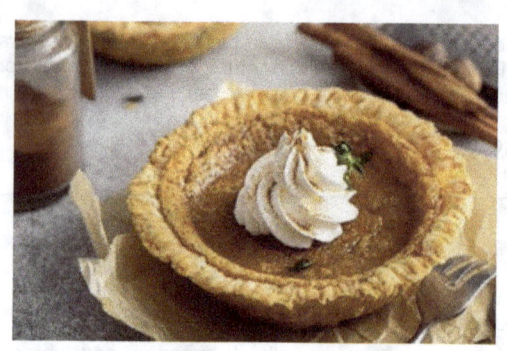

While Rwandan cuisine is primarily known for its savory dishes, the country also offers some delectable desserts. One such dessert is the Banana Cake, made with ripe bananas and often flavored with cinnamon or nutmeg, offering a delightful balance of sweetness and warmth.

INGREDIENTS

- 2 cups mashed sweet potatoes
- 1 cup granulated sugar
- 1/2 cup milk
- 2 eggs, beaten
- 2 tablespoons melted butter
- 1 teaspoon vanilla extract
- 1/4 teaspoon salt 1 pre-made pie crust1/4 teaspoon ground nutme
- 1/2 teaspoon ground cinnamon

DIRECTIONS

1. Preheat your oven to 375°F (190°C).
2. In a large bowl, combine the mashed sweet potatoes, sugar, milk, beaten eggs, melted butter, vanilla extract, cinnamon, nutmeg, and salt. Mix well until smooth and creamy.
3. Roll out the pre-made pie crust and line a pie dish with it.
4. Pour the sweet potato mixture into the pie crust, spreading it evenly.
5. Bake in the preheated oven for about 45-50 minutes, or until the filling is set and the crust is golden brown.
6. Remove from the oven and let the pie cool before serving. Slice and enjoy this delicious Rwandan sweet potato pie!

ASIA

PIES & COBBLERS

Coffee Pie —Vietnam

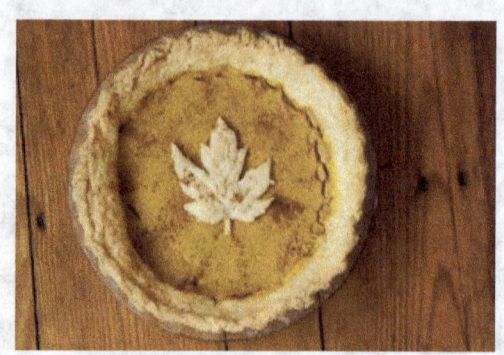

Vietnamese cuisine is renowned for its delicate and vibrant flavors, and its desserts are no exception. Try the famous Che, a sweet soup made with various ingredients such as beans, coconut milk, and tapioca pearls, or indulge in a Banh Chuoi Nuong, a delicious banana cake and irresistible coffee pie

INGREDIENTS

- 1 pre-made chocolate cookie crust
- 1 cup strong brewed Vietnamese coffee, cooled
- 1 cup heavy cream
- 1/2 cup sweetened condensed milk
- 1 tablespoon gelatin powder
- Whipped cream and chocolate shavings for garnish

DIRECTIONS

1. In a small bowl, dissolve the gelatin powder in 1/4 cup of cold water. Let it sit for a few minutes to bloom.
2. In a saucepan, heat the brewed Vietnamese coffee over medium heat until warm. Do not boil.
3. In a separate bowl, whisk together the heavy cream and sweetened condensed milk until well combined.
4. Stir the bloomed gelatin into the warm coffee until fully dissolved.
5. Gradually whisk the coffee mixture into the cream mixture until smooth and well incorporated.
6. Pour the coffee mixture into the pre-made chocolate cookie crust.
7. Refrigerate the pie for at least 4 hours, or until set.
8. Before serving, garnish with whipped cream and chocolate shavings.
9. Slice and enjoy this indulgent Vietnamese coffee pie!

PIES & COBBLERS

Pineapple Cobbler — Taiwan

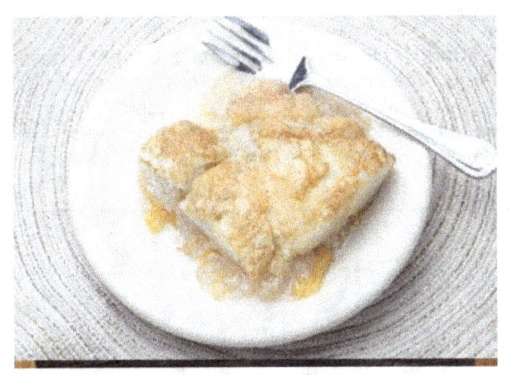

Taiwan is a haven for dessert lovers. The country is famous for its night markets, where you can find a variety of sweet treats. Try the iconic Bubble Tea, a refreshing drink with tapioca pearls, or sample the Pineapple Cake, a buttery pastry filled with sweet pineapple jam.

INGREDIENTS

- 2 cups fresh pineapple, diced
- 1/2 cup granulated sugar
- 1 tablespoon cornstarch
- 1 tablespoon lemon juice ⊠ 1 cup all-purpose flour
- 1/4 cup granulated sugar
- 1 teaspoon baking powder
- 1/4 teaspoon salt
- 1/2 cup unsalted butter, cold and diced
- 1/4 cup milk
- 1/2 teaspoon vanilla extract

DIRECTIONS

1. Preheat your oven to 375°F (190°C).
2. In a mixing bowl, combine the diced pineapple, granulated sugar, cornstarch, and lemon juice. Toss gently to coat the pineapple evenly, and set aside.
3. In a separate bowl, whisk together the flour, granulated sugar, baking powder, and salt.
4. Add the cold diced butter to the flour mixture and use a pastry cutter or your fingertips to cut the butter into the flour until it resembles coarse crumbs.
5. Stir in the milk and vanilla extract until the dough just comes together.
6. Transfer the pineapple mixture to a baking dish. Drop a spoonful of the dough evenly over the pineapple.
7. Bake the cobbler in the preheated oven for about 3540 minutes, or until the topping is golden brown and the pineapple is bubbly.
8. Remove from the oven and let the cobbler cool slightly before serving. Serve warm and enjoy the tropical flavors of this Taiwanese pineapple cobbler!

PIES & COBBLERS

Egg Custard Tart — Hong Kong

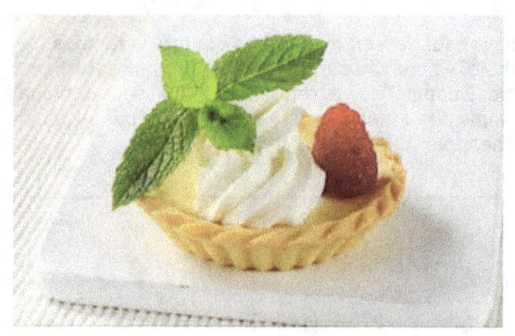

Hong Kong offers a blend of traditional Cantonese desserts and international influences. Don't miss out on the iconic Egg Tart, a flaky pastry filled with smooth egg custard, or indulge in the classic Mango Pomelo Sago, a refreshing dessert made with fresh mango, pomelo, and sago pearls.

INGREDIENTS

- 1 package of pre-made puff pastry dough
- 4 egg yolks
- 1/2 cup granulated sugar
- 1 cup milk
- 1/2 teaspoon vanilla extract

DIRECTIONS

1. Preheat your oven to 375°F (190°C).
2. Roll out the pre-made puff pastry dough and cut it into circles to fit a muffin tin.
3. Line each muffin cup with the puff pastry circles, pressing gently to fit.
4. In a mixing bowl, whisk together the egg yolks and sugar until well combined.
5. In a saucepan, heat the milk over medium heat until it comes to a simmer.
6. Gradually pour the simmering milk into the egg yolk mixture, whisking
7. Constantly to prevent the eggs from curdling. 7. Stir in the vanilla extract.
8. Pour the custard mixture into the prepared puff pastry cups, filling them about 3/4 full.
9. Bake in the preheated oven for about 15-20 minutes, or until the custard is set and the pastry is golden brown.
10. Remove from the oven and let the tarts cool before serving. Enjoy these delightful Hong Kong egg custard tarts!

Australia & Oceania

PIES & COBBLERS

Coconut Cream Pie — Solomon Islands

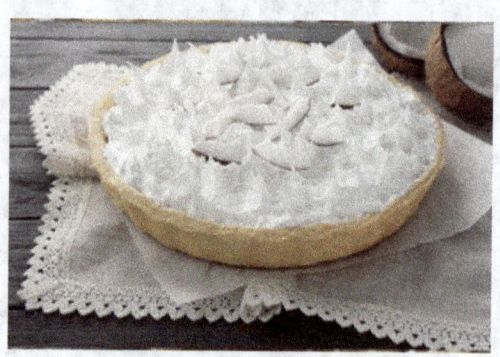

The Solomon Islands boast a tropical paradise with a rich culinary heritage. When it comes to desserts, the islands offer a delightful array of tropical fruits. Enjoy a refreshing Papaya Boat, where the fruit is hollowed out and filled with other fruits like bananas and passion fruit.

INGREDIENTS

- 1 1/2 cups graham cracker crumbs
- 1/4 cup granulated sugar ⬚ 1/2 cup unsalted butter, melted

For the filling:
- 1 can (14 oz) coconut milk
- 1 cup whole milk
- 3/4 cup granulated sugar
- 1/3 cup cornstarch
- 4 egg yolks
- 1 teaspoon vanilla extract
- Whipped cream and toasted coconut flakes for garnish

DIRECTIONS

1. Preheat your oven to 375°F (190°C).
2. In a mixing bowl, combine the graham cracker crumbs, granulated sugar, and melted butter for the crust. Stir until the mixture resembles wet sand.
3. Press the crumb mixture into a pie dish, forming an even crust along the bottom and sides.
4. Bake the crust in the preheated oven for about 8-10 minutes, or until golden brown. Remove from the oven and let it cool.
5. In a saucepan, heat the coconut milk and whole milk over medium heat until steaming, but not boiling.
6. In a separate bowl, whisk together the granulated sugar, cornstarch, and egg yolks until well combined.
7. Slowly pour the hot milk mixture into the egg mixture, whisking constantly.
8. Return the mixture to the saucepan and cook over medium heat, stirring constantly, until thickened and smooth. Finally, add vanilla essence or extract. Turn off the flame.
9. Pour the filling into the baked crust and smooth the top. Refrigerate the pie for at least 4 hours, or until set.
10. Before serving, garnish with whipped cream and toasted coconut flakes.
11. Slice and enjoy this creamy and tropical Solomon Islands coconut cream pie!

PIES & COBBLERS

Banana Cream Pie — American Samoa

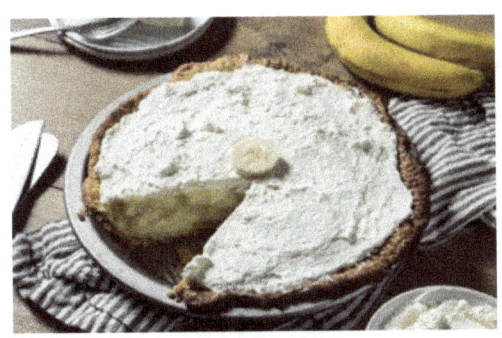

American Samoa's desserts often feature the flavors of coconut and banana. Try the delicious Panikeke, which are fluffy Samoan pancakes, or the Fausi, a rich coconut bread pudding.

INGREDIENTS

- 1 1/2 cups graham cracker crumbs
- 1/4 cup granulated sugar ⊠ 1/2 cup unsalted butter, melted

For the filling:

- 3 ripe bananas, sliced
- 1 cup heavy cream
- 1/2 cup whole milk
- 1/2 cup granulated sugar
- 1/4 cup cornstarch
- 4 egg yolks
- 1 teaspoon vanilla extract
- Whipped cream and banana slices for garnish

DIRECTIONS

1. Preheat your oven to 375°F (190°C).
2. In a mixing bowl, combine the graham cracker crumbs, granulated sugar, and melted butter for the crust. Stir until the mixture resembles wet sand.
3. Press the crumb mixture into a pie dish, forming an even crust along the bottom and sides.
4. Bake the crust in the preheated oven for about 8-10 minutes, or until golden brown. Remove from the oven and let it cool.
5. Arrange the sliced bananas over the cooled crust.
6. In a saucepan, heat the heavy cream and whole milk over medium heat until steaming, but not boiling.
7. In a separate bowl, whisk together the granulated sugar, cornstarch, and egg yolks until well combined.
8. Slowly pour the hot milk mixture into the egg mixture, whisking constantly.
9. Return the mixture to the saucepan and cook over medium heat, stirring constantly, until thickened and smooth.
10. Remove from heat and stir in the vanilla extract.
11. Pour the filling over the sliced bananas in the crust and smooth the top.
12. Refrigerate the pie for at least 4 hours, or until set.
13. Before serving, garnish with whipped cream and banana slices.
14. Slice and enjoy this luscious American Samoa banana cream pie!

PIES & COBBLERS

Coconut Pie — Tokelau

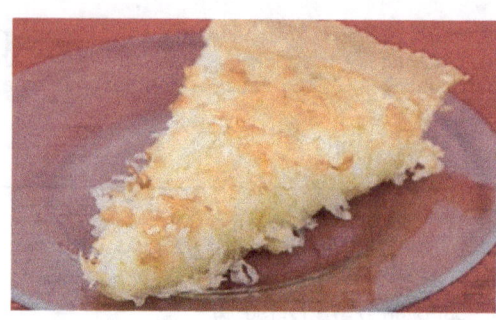

Tokelau, a small island territory of New Zealand, offers traditional Polynesian desserts. One such delight is the Tulikiga, a sweet coconut dessert made from grated coconut and sugar.

INGREDIENTS

- 1 1/2 cups all-purpose flour
- 1/4 cup granulated sugar
- 1/2 teaspoon salt
- 1/2 cup unsalted butter, cold and diced
- 2-3 tablespoons ice water

For the filling:

- 2 cups shredded coconut ▢ 1/2 cup granulated sugar
- 3 tablespoons all-purpose flour
- 1/4 teaspoon salt
- 1 cup coconut milk
- 1/2 cup whole milk
- 1 teaspoon vanilla extract

DIRECTIONS

1. Preheat your oven to 375°F (190°C).
2. In a mixing bowl, combine the flour, sugar, and salt for the crust. Add the cold diced butter and use a pastry cutter or your fingertips to cut the butter into the flour until it resembles coarse crumbs.
3. Gradually add the ice water, mixing until the dough comes together. Shape the dough into a ball, wrap it in plastic wrap, and refrigerate for 30 minutes.
4. Roll out the chilled dough on a lightly floured surface and fit it into a 9-inch pie dish. Trim any excess dough from the edges and crimp them decoratively.
5. In a separate bowl, combine the shredded coconut, granulated sugar, flour, and salt for the filling.
6. In a saucepan, heat the coconut milk and whole milk over medium heat until steaming, but not boiling.
7. Slowly pour the hot milk mixture into the coconut mixture, stirring constantly.
8. Stir in the vanilla extract until well combined.
9. Pour the filling into the prepared crust, spreading it evenly.
10. Bake in the preheated oven for about 25-30 minutes, or until the filling is set and the crust is golden brown.
11. Remove from the oven and let the pie.
12. Cool before serving.
13. Once cooled, slice and enjoy this delicious Tokelauan coconut pie, which captures the rich and tropical flavors of the region.

EUROPE

PIES & COBBLERS

Pastel de Nata (Custard Tart) —Portugal

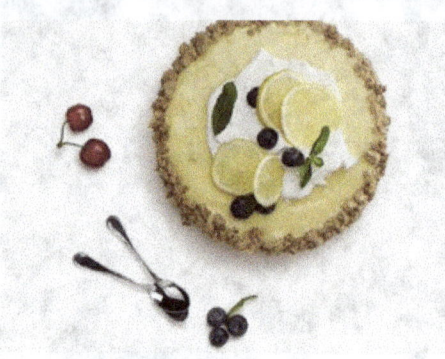

Portuguese desserts are known for their rich flavors and use of traditional ingredients. Indulge in the iconic Pasteis de Nata, creamy custard tarts with a crispy pastry shell, or savor the deliciously moist Pão de Ló, a traditional Portuguese sponge cake.

INGREDIENTS

- 2 sheets puff pastry, thawed
- Flour for dusting
- For the custard filling:
- 2 cups mil
- 1 cinnamon stick
- Zest of 1 lemon
- 6 egg yolks
- 1/2 cup granulated sugar
- 2 tablespoons all-purpose flour
- Powdered sugar and ground cinnamon for dusting

DIRECTIONS

1. Preheat your oven to 425°F (220°C).
2. On a lightly floured surface, roll out the puff pastry sheets to a thin rectangle.
3. Starting from one end, roll the pastry tightly into a log shape. Cut the log into 12 equal slices.
4. Flatten each slice with the palm of your hand and press them into the cups of a muffin tin, lining the bottom and sides to form tart shells.
5. In a saucepan, heat the milk, cinnamon stick, and lemon zest over medium heat until it comes to a simmer. Remove from heat and let it steep for 10 minutes.
6. In a mixing bowl, whisk together the egg yolks, granulated sugar, and flour until smooth.
7. Remove the cinnamon stick and lemon zest from the milk mixture.
8. Slowly pour the milk mixture into the egg yolk mixture, whisking constantly.
9. Place the muffin tin with the pastry shells on a baking sheet and carefully pour the custard filling into each shell, filling them about 3/4 full.
10. Bake in the preheated oven for about 15-20 minutes, or until the custard is set and the pastry is golden brown. Remove from the oven and let the pastéis de nata cool in the tin for a few minutes before transferring them to a wire rack to cool completely.
11. Before serving, dust the pastéis de nata with powdered sugar and ground cinnamon.
12. Enjoy these delicious and iconic Portuguese custard tarts!

PIES & COBBLERS

Dobos Torte (Layered Sponge Cake) — Hungary

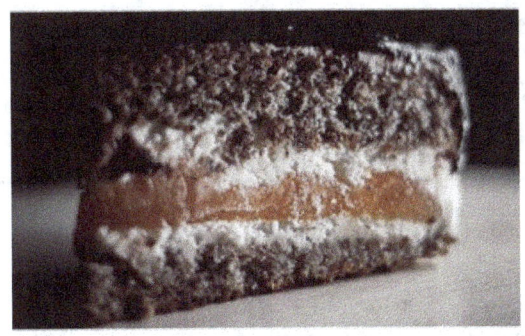

Hungarian desserts are a blend of sweetness and elegance. Try the famous Dobos Torte, a layered cake with chocolate buttercream and caramel, or enjoy the decadent SomlóiGaluska, a trifle-like dessert made with sponge cake, chocolate sauce, and whipped cream.

INGREDIENTS

- 6 large eggs, separated
- 1 cup granulated sugar
- 1 teaspoon vanilla extract
- 1 cup all-purpose flour (Remove 4 tabspoon flour and add 4tabspooncocopowder
- 1/4 teaspoon salt
- For the chocolate buttercream:
- 1 cup unsalted butter, softened
- 1 1/2 cups powdered sugar
- 4 ounces semisweet chocolate, melted and cooled ☒ 1 teaspoon vanilla extract ☒ For the caramel topping:
- 1 cup granulated sugar
- 1/4 cup water
- Whipped cream and caramel drizzle for garnish

DIRECTIONS

1. Preheat your oven to 350°F (175°C). Grease and flour a 9-inch round cake pan.
2. In a mixing bowl, beat the egg yolks, granulated sugar, and vanilla extract until pale and creamy.
3. In a separate bowl, whisk together the flour and salt.
4. Gradually add the flour mixture to the egg yolk mixture, mixing until just combined.
5. In another clean bowl, beat the egg whites until stiff peaks form.
6. Gently fold the beaten egg whites into the batter until incorporated. Pour the batter into the prepared cake pan and spread it evenly.
7. Bake in the preheated oven for about 25-30 minutes, or until a toothpick inserted into the center comes out clean. Remove from the oven and let the cake cool in the pan for a few minutes before transferring it to a wire rack to cool completely.
8. In a mixing bowl, beat the softened butter until creamy. Gradually add the powdered sugar and continue to beat until light and fluffy.
9. Stir in the melted chocolate and vanilla extract until well combined. Cut the cooled sponge cake into 6 equal layers.
10. Spread a thin layer of chocolate buttercream on top of each layer, stacking them one on top of the other. For the caramel topping, heat the granulated sugar and water in a saucepan over medium heat until the sugar dissolves and turns into a golden caramel color.
11. Remove from heat and quickly pour the caramel over the top layer of the cake, allowing it to drip down the sides. Let the caramel set and cool completely before decorating with whipped cream and a drizzle of caramel.
12. Slice and enjoy this iconic Hungarian Dobos Torte with its rich layers of sponge cake, chocolate buttercream, and caramel topping.

PIES & COBBLERS

Lingonberry Pie —Finland

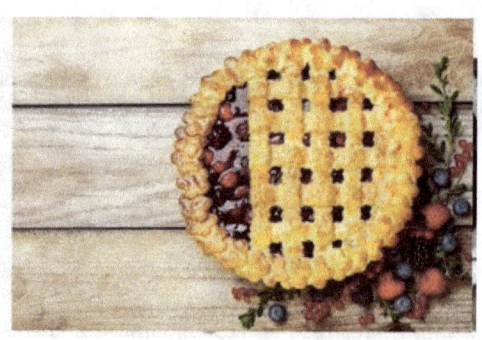

Finnish desserts often highlight the flavors of berries and cardamom. Sample the Runeberg Torte, a traditional almond and raspberry tart, or savor the must-try Vispipuuro, a delightful berry semolina porridge topped with vanilla sauce.

INGREDIENTS

- 2 1/2 cups all-purpose flour
- 1/2 teaspoon salt
- 1 cup unsalted butter, cold and diced
- 1/2 cup ice water

For the filling:
- 4 cups fresh or frozen lingonberries
- 1 cup granulated sugar
- 2 tablespoons cornstarch
- 1 tablespoon lemon juice

DIRECTIONS

1. Preheat your oven to 375°F (190°C).
2. In a mixing bowl, whisk together the flour and salt for the crust. Add the cold diced butter and use a pastry cutter or your fingertips to cut the butter into the flour until it resembles coarse crumbs.
3. Gradually add the ice water, mixing until the dough comes together. Shape the dough into a ball, wrap it in plastic wrap, and refrigerate for 30 minutes.
4. Roll out half of the chilled dough on a lightly floured surface and fit it into a 9-inch pie dish. Trim any excess dough from the edges.
5. In a separate bowl, combine the lingonberries, granulated sugar, cornstarch, and lemon juice for the filling. Mix well to coat the lingonberries evenly.
6. Pour the lingonberry mixture into the prepared crust, spreading it out evenly.
7. Roll out the remaining half of the chilled dough and place it over the filling, sealing the edges with the bottom crust. Cut a few small slits on the top crust to allow steam to escape during baking.
8. Optional: You can brush the top crust with an egg wash (1 beaten egg mixed with a tablespoon of water) for a shiny golden finish.
9. Place the pie on a baking sheet and bake in the preheated oven for about 40-45 minutes, or until the crust is golden brown and the filling is bubbling.
10. Remove from the oven and let the pie cool before serving.
11. Slice and enjoy this delicious Finnish lingonberry pie, which showcases the tart and vibrant flavors of the beloved lingonberries.

CARIBBEAN

PIES & COBBLERS

Nutmeg Cake—Grenada

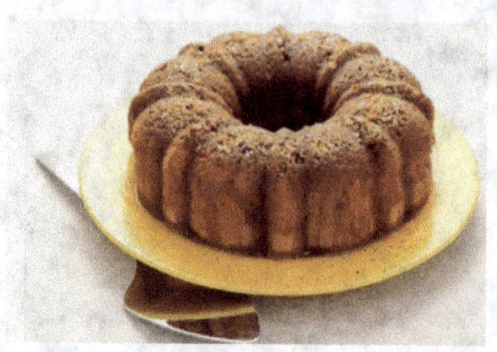

Grenada, known as the "Spice Island," infuses its desserts with aromatic spices such as nutmeg and cinnamon. Don't miss out on the Nutmeg Ice Cream, a creamy treat flavored with Grenada's famous nutmeg spice.

INGREDIENTS

- 2 cups all-purpose flour
- 2 teaspoons baking powder
- 1/2 teaspoon salt
- 1 teaspoon ground nutmeg
- 1 cup unsalted butter, softened
- 1 1/2 cups granulated sugar
- 4 eggs
- 1 cup milk
- 1 teaspoon vanilla extract
- Powdered sugar for dusting

DIRECTIONS

1. Preheat your oven to 350°F (175°C). Grease and flour a 9-inch round cake pan.
2. In a mixing bowl, whisk together the flour, baking powder, salt, and ground nutmeg.
3. In another bowl, Mix butter and sugar with a beater until you get a light and fluffy mixture.
4. Beat in the eggs, one at a time, until well combined.
5. Add the dry ingredients to the butter mixture alternately with the milk, beginning and ending with the dry ingredients. Mix until just combined.
6. Stir in the vanilla extract.
7. Pour the batter into the prepared cake pan and spread it evenly.
8. Bake in the preheated oven for about 30-35 minutes, or until a toothpick inserted into the center comes out clean.
9. Remove from the oven and let the cake cool in the pan for a few minutes before transferring it to a wire rack to cool completely.
10. Dust the cooled nutmeg cake with powdered sugar before serving.
11. Slice and savor the warm and aromatic flavors of this Grenadian nutmeg cake.

PIES & COBBLERS

Leches Cake — Dominican Republic

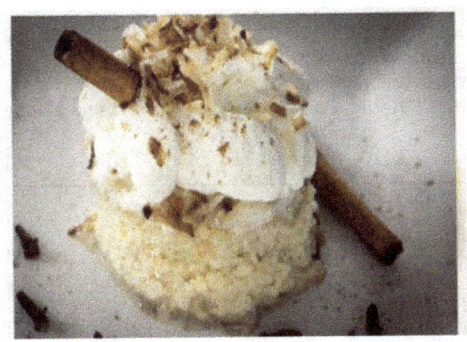

Dominican desserts feature a fusion of African, Spanish, and indigenous Taino flavors. Indulge in the popular TresLeches Cake, a moist sponge cake soaked in three types of milk, or enjoy the sweet and buttery BizcochoDominicano, a traditional Dominican cake.

INGREDIENTS

- 1 1/2 cups all-purpose flour
- 1 1/2 teaspoons baking powder
- 1/4 teaspoon salt
- 4 large eggs
- 1 cup granulated sugar
- 1/2 cup unsalted butter, melted
- 1 teaspoon vanilla extract
- For the Tresleches mixture:
- 1 can (14 oz) sweetened condensed milk
- 1 can (12 oz) evaporated milk
- 1 cup whole milk
- For the whipped cream topping:
- 2 cups heavy cream
- 1/4 cup granulated sugar
- 1 teaspoon vanilla extract

DIRECTIONS

1. Preheat your oven to 350°F (175°C). Grease and flour a 9x13-inch baking dish.
2. In a mixing bowl, whisk together the flour, baking powder, and salt for the cake.
3. In a separate bowl, beat the eggs and granulated sugar together until light and fluffy.
4. Gradually add the melted butter and vanilla extract to the egg mixture, mixing well.
5. Add the dry ingredients to the egg mixture and mix until just combined.
6. Pour the batter into the prepared baking dish and spread it evenly.
7. Bake in the preheated oven for about 25-30 minutes, or until a toothpick inserted into the center comes out clean.
8. Remove from the oven and let the cake cool in the dish for a few minutes.
9. In a mixing bowl, whisk together the sweetened condensed milk, evaporated milk, and whole milk for the tres leches mixture.
10. Use a fork or skewer to poke holes all over the surface of the warm cake.
11. Slowly pour the tres leches mixture over the cake, allowing it to soak into the holes and absorb the milk.
12. Cover the cake and refrigerate for at least 2 hours, or overnight, to allow the cake to absorb the milk mixture.
13. In a mixing bowl, beat the heavy cream, granulated sugar, and vanilla extract together until stiff peaks form.
14. Spread the whipped cream over the chilled cake.
15. Slice and indulge in this decadent Dominican TresLeches Cake, with its moist sponge cake soaked in a luscious milk mixture and topped with fluffy whipped cream.

PIES & COBBLERS

Guava Duff – Bahamas

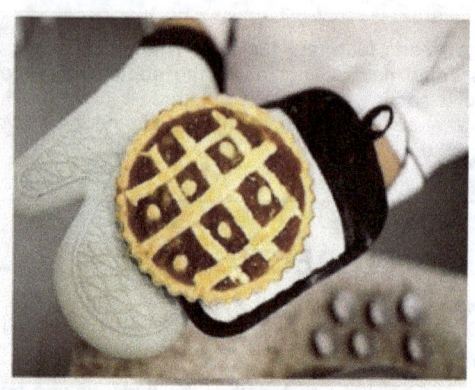

Finnish desserts often highlight the flavors of berries and cardamom. Sample the Runeberg Torte, a traditional almond and raspberry tart, or savor the must-try Vispipuuro, a delightful berry semolina porridge topped with vanilla sauce.

INGREDIENTS

- 2 cups all-purpose flour
- 2 teaspoons baking powder
- 1/2 teaspoon salt
- 1/4 cup granulated sugar
- 1/2 cup unsalted butter, cold and diced
- 2/3 cup milk ⊠ 1 teaspoon vanilla extract ⊠ For the guava filling:
- 2 cups guava pulp (available in canned or frozen form)
- 1/2 cup granulated sugar ⊠ 1/4 teaspoon ground cinnamon ⊠ For the rum sauce:
- 1 cup unsalted butter
- 1 cup granulated sugar
- 1/2 cup heavy cream
- 1/4 cup rum (optional)
- Whipped cream for serving (optional)

DIRECTIONS

1. Preheat your oven to 350°F (175°C).
2. In a mixing bowl, whisk together the flour, baking powder, salt, and granulated sugar for the dough.
3. Add the cold diced butter to the flour mixture and use a pastry cutter or your fingertips to cut the butter into the flour until it resembles coarse crumbs. 4. Gradually add the milk and vanilla extract to the dough, mixing until it comes together.
4. On a lightly floured surface, roll out the dough into a large rectangle, about 1/4 inch thick.
5. In a separate bowl, combine the guava pulp, granulated sugar, and ground cinnamon for the filling. Mix well to combine.
6. Spread the guava filling evenly over the rolled-out dough.
7. Carefully roll up the dough, starting from one of the long sides, to form a log.
8. Place the guava-filled dough log into a greased baking dish.
9. Bake in the preheated oven for about 45-50 minutes, or until the duff is golden brown and cooked through.
10. While the duff is baking, prepare the rum sauce.
11. Melt the butter in a saucepan on medium heat
12. Stir in the granulated sugar and cook until dissolved.
13. Stir in the heavy cream and continue to cook until the sauce thickens slightly. Remove the saucepan from heat and stir in the rum, if using.
14. Once the guava duff is done baking, remove it from the oven and let it cool slightly. Serve slices of the warm guava duff drizzled with the rum sauce.
15. Optionally, you can also top the duff with a dollop of whipped cream.
16. Enjoy this delightful Bahamian dessert, with its sweet guava filling and decadent rum sauce!

South America & Latin America

PIES & COBBLERS

Chilean Apple Cobbler — Chile

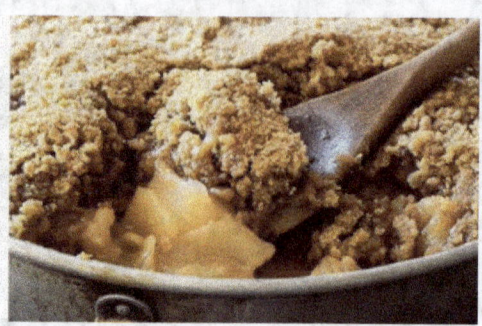

Chilean desserts highlight the country's agricultural abundance. Sample the delicious Leche Asada, a baked milk custard dessert, or enjoy the comforting Torta de Mil Hojas, a layered puff pastry cake filled with dulce de leche and topped with powdered sugar.

INGREDIENTS

- 4 cups sliced apples
- 1/2 cup granulated sugar
  - 1 tablespoon lemon juice
  - 1 teaspoon ground cinnamon

For the topping:
- 1 cup all-purpose flour
- 1/2 cup granulated sugar
- 1 teaspoon baking powder
- 1/4 teaspoon salt
- 1/2 cup unsalted butter, cold and diced
- 1/4 cup milk
- 1 teaspoon vanilla extract

DIRECTIONS

1. Preheat your oven to 375°F (190°C).
2. In a mixing bowl, combine the sliced apples, granulated sugar, lemon juice, and ground cinnamon for the filling. Toss gently to coat the apples evenly.
3. Transfer the apple mixture to a baking dish.
4. In a separate bowl, whisk together the flour, granulated sugar, baking powder, and salt for the topping.
5. Add the cold diced butter to the flour mixture and use a pastry cutter or your fingertips to cut the butter into the flour until it resembles coarse crumbs.
6. Stir in the milk and vanilla extract until the dough just comes together.
7. Drop a spoonful of the dough evenly over the apple mixture.
8. Bake the cobbler in the preheated oven for about 3035 minutes, or until the topping is golden brown and the apples are bubbling.
9. Remove from the oven and let the cobbler cool slightly before serving. Serve warm and enjoy the comforting flavors of this Chilean apple cobbler.

PIES & COBBLERS

Dutch Apple Pie — Bonaire

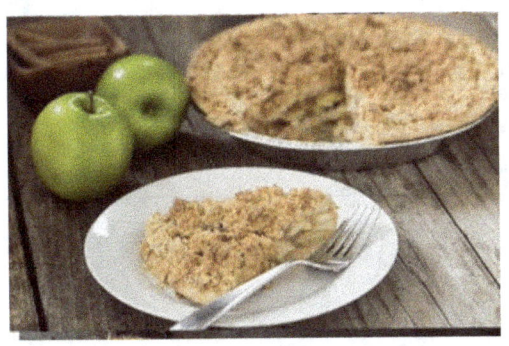

Bonaire, a Dutch Caribbean island, offers delightful sweet treats influenced by Dutch cuisine. Try the Poffertjes, small fluffy pancakes served with powdered sugar and butter, or savor the traditional Bolo di Cashupete, a rich cashew cake.

INGREDIENTS

- 2 1/2 cups all-purpose flour
- 1 teaspoon salt
- 1 cup unsalted butter, cold and diced
- 1/4 cup ice water

For the filling:
- 6 cups sliced apples
- 1/2 cup granulated sugar
- 1/4 cup all-purpose flour
- 1 teaspoon ground cinnamon
- 1/4 teaspoon ground nutmeg
- 1 tablespoon lemon juice For the crumb topping:
- 1 cup all-purpose flour
- 1/2 cup granulated sugar
- 1/2 cup unsalted butter, melted

DIRECTIONS

1. Preheat your oven to 375°F (190°C).
2. In a mixing bowl, whisk together the flour and salt for the crust. Add the cold diced butter and use a pastry cutter or your fingertips to cut the butter into the flour until it resembles coarse crumbs.
3. Gradually add the ice water, mixing until the dough comes together. Shape the dough into a ball, wrap it in plastic wrap, and refrigerate for 30 minutes.
4. Roll out half of the chilled dough on a lightly floured surface and fit it into a 9-inch pie dish. Trim any excess dough from the edges.
5. In a separate bowl, combine the sliced apples, granulated sugar, flour, ground cinnamon, ground nutmeg, and lemon juice for the filling. Mix well to coat the apples evenly.
6. Pour the apple filling into the prepared crust, spreading it out evenly.
7. Roll out the remaining half of the chilled dough and place it over the filling, sealing the edges with the bottom crust. Cut a few small slits on the top crust to allow steam to escape during baking.
8. In a separate bowl, combine the flour, granulated sugar, and melted butter for the crumb topping. Mix until crumbly.
9. Sprinkle the crumb topping over the pie, covering the entire surface.
10. Bake in the preheated oven for about 50-60 minutes, or until the crust is golden brown and the apples are tender.
11. Remove from the oven and let the pie cool before serving.
12. Slice and enjoy this classic Dutch apple pie, with its buttery crust, sweet apple filling, and crunchy crumb topping.

PIES & COBBLERS

Pineapple Cobbler — Costa Rico

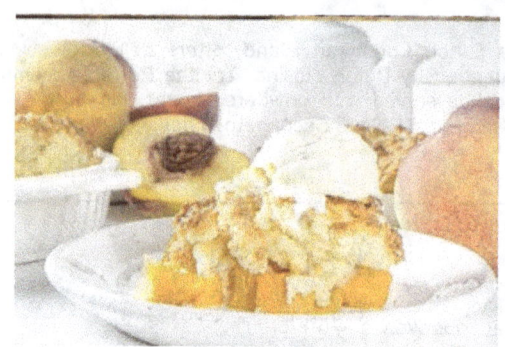

Costa Rican desserts feature a variety of tropical fruits and flavors. Indulge in the classic TresLeches Cake, a favorite among locals, or enjoy the refreshing Helado de Sorbetera, a traditional Costa Rican ice cream made with fresh fruit.

INGREDIENTS

- 4 cups fresh pineapple chunks
- 1/2 cup granulated sugar ☒ 2 tablespoons cornstarch ☒ 1 tablespoon lemon juice For the topping:
- 1 cup all-purpose flour
- 1/2 cup granulated sugar
- 1 teaspoon baking powder
- 1/4 teaspoon salt
- 1/2 cup unsalted butter, cold and diced
- 1/4 cup milk 1 teaspoon vanilla extract

DIRECTIONS

1. Preheat your oven to 375°F (190°C).
2. In a mixing bowl, combine the pineapple chunks, granulated sugar, cornstarch, and lemon juice for the filling. Toss gently to coat the pineapple evenly.
3. Transfer the pineapple mixture to a baking dish.
4. In a separate bowl, whisk together the flour, granulated sugar, baking powder, and salt for the topping.
5. Add the cold diced butter to the flour mixture and use a pastry cutter or your fingertips to cut the butter into the flour until it resembles coarse crumbs.
6. Stir in the milk and vanilla extract until the dough just comes together.
7. Drop spoonfuls of the dough evenly over the pineapple mixture.
8. Bake the cobbler in the preheated oven for about 3035 minutes, or until the topping is golden brown and the pineapple is bubbling.
9. Remove from the oven and let the cobbler cool slightly before serving. Serve warm and enjoy the tropical flavors of this Costa Rican pineapple cobbler.

NORTH AMERICA

PIES & COBBLERS

US Biscochitos — New Mexico

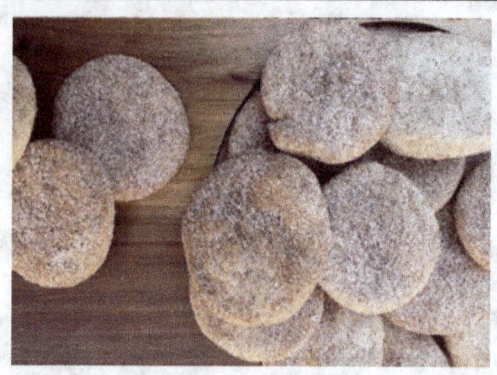

New Mexican desserts blend indigenous, Spanish, and Mexican influences. Savor the iconic Biscochitos, buttery cinnamon, and anise-flavored cookies, or try the fluffy and moist Sopaipillas, fried pastries served with honey

INGREDIENTS

- 3 cups all-purpose flour
- 1 1/2 teaspoons baking powder
- 1/2 teaspoon salt
- 1 cup unsalted butter, softened
- 1 cup granulated sugar
- 2 large eggs
- 1 teaspoon anise extract
- 1/4 cup brandy or rum (optional)
- 1/4 cup milk (if needed)
- 1/2 cup granulated sugar mixed with 1 tablespoon ground cinnamon, for rolling

DIRECTIONS

1. Preheat your oven to 350°F (175°C).
2. In a mixing bowl, whisk together the flour, baking powder, and salt.
3. Take a separate bowl and mix the softened butter and granulated sugar until they are creamed together, resulting in a light and fluffy consistency.
4. Beat in the eggs, one at a time, followed by the anise extract and brandy or rum (if using).
5. Gradually add the flour mixture to the butter mixture, mixing until a dough forms. If the dough is too dry, add milk, a tablespoon at a time, until it comes together.
6. Divide the dough into two portions and wrap each portion in plastic wrap. Refrigerate for about 30 minutes to firm up.
7. On a lightly floured surface, roll out one portion of the dough to about 1/4-inch thickness. Use cookie cutters to cut out shapes, traditionally anise-flavored circles or stars.
8. Place the cut-out cookies on a baking sheet lined with parchment paper, spacing them about 1 inch apart.
9. Bake in the preheated oven for about 10-12 minutes, or until the edges are lightly golden.
10. Remove the cookies from the oven and let them cool on the baking sheet for a few minutes before transferring them to a wire rack.
11. While the cookies are still warm, roll them in the cinnamon-sugar mixture to coat.
12. Repeat the process with the remaining portion of the dough.
13. Serve and savor the delightful flavors of these traditional New Mexican Biscochitos, perfect for holiday feasting!

PIES & COBBLERS

Butter Tart — Toronto, Canada

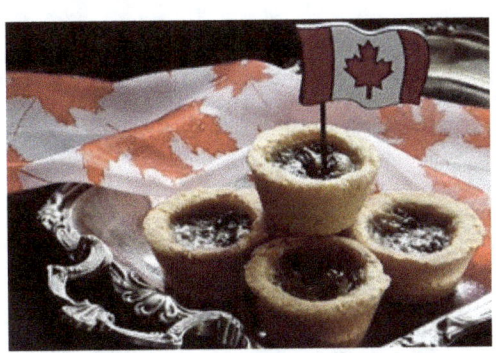

Toronto offers a multicultural food scene, including a wide range of desserts. Sample the decadent Butter Tart, a sweet pastry filled with a gooey and buttery caramelized filling, or enjoy the classic Nanaimo Bars, layered bars with a creamy custard filling.

INGREDIENTS

- Ingredients: For the pastry:
- 1 1/4 cups all-purpose flour
- 1/4 teaspoon salt
- 1/2 cup unsalted butter, cold and diced
- 2-3 tablespoons ice water

For the filling:
- 1/2 cup unsalted butter, melted
- 1 cup brown sugar
- 1/4 cup maple syrup
- 1/4 cup corn syrup
- 2 large eggs
- 1 teaspoon vanilla extract
- 1/4 teaspoon salt
- 1 cup raisins or pecans (optional)

DIRECTIONS

1. In a mixing bowl, whisk together the flour and salt for the pastry.
2. Add the cold diced butter to the flour mixture and use a pastry cutter or your fingertips to cut the butter into the flour until it resembles coarse crumbs.
3. Gradually add the ice water, mixing until the dough comes together. Shape the dough into a ball, wrap it in plastic wrap, and refrigerate for 30 minutes.
4. Preheat your oven to 375°F (190°C).
5. On a lightly floured surface, roll out the chilled dough and cut it into rounds to fit a muffin tin.
6. Press each round into the greased muffin tin, forming a small pastry cup.
7. In a mixing bowl, combine the melted butter, brown sugar, maple syrup, corn syrup, eggs, vanilla extract, and salt for the filling. Mix well to combine.
8. If desired, add raisins or pecans to the filling mixture.
9. Spoon the filling into the prepared pastry cups, filling them about 3/4 full.
10. Bake in the preheated oven for about 15-20 minutes, or until the pastry is golden brown and the filling is set.
11. Remove from the oven and let the butter tarts cool in the tin for a few minutes before transferring them to a wire rack to cool completely.
12. Serve the butter tarts at room temperature. Enjoy these sweet and gooey treats that are beloved in Toronto!

PIES & COBBLERS

Mexican Flan — Chichen Itza (Mexico)

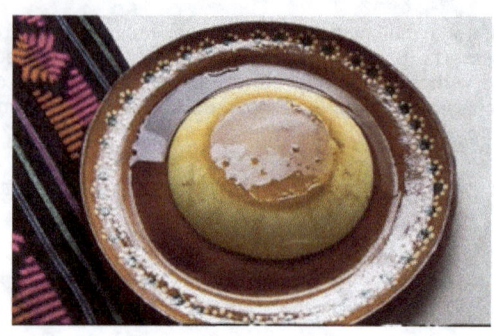

Chichen Itza, a historical site in Mexico, is famous for its rich culinary heritage. While not known for its desserts, you can find traditional Mexican sweets such as Mexican Flan, a creamy caramel custard, which is often enjoyed as a sweet ending to a meal.

INGREDIENTS

- 1 cup granulated sugar
- 4 large eggs
- 1 can (14 ounces) of sweetened condensed milk
- 1 can (12 ounces) of evaporated milk
- 1 teaspoon vanilla extract
- Pinch of salt

DIRECTIONS

1. Preheat your oven to 350°F (175°C).
2. In a saucepan, melt the granulated sugar over medium heat, stirring constantly until it caramelizes and turns golden brown.
3. Quickly pour the caramelized sugar into a round baking dish, tilting the dish to coat the bottom and sides evenly. Set aside to cool and harden.
4. In a mixing bowl, whisk together the eggs, sweetened condensed milk, evaporated milk, vanilla extract, and salt until well combined.
5. Pour the egg mixture into the caramel-coated baking dish.
6. Place the baking dish in a larger roasting pan and create a water bath by filling the roasting pan with hot water until it reaches halfway up the sides of the baking dish.
7. Carefully transfer the roasting pan with the water bath and the flan mixture to the preheated oven.
8. Bake for about 50-60 minutes, or until the flan is set but still slightly jiggly in the center.
9. Remove the baking dish from the water bath and let it cool to room temperature.
10. Once cooled, cover the baking dish with plastic wrap and refrigerate for at least 4 hours or overnight to allow the flan to firm up.
11. To serve, run a knife around the edges of the baking dish to loosen the flan. Place a serving plate upside down on top of the dish and flip it over to release the flan onto the plate. The caramel sauce will flow over the flan.
12. Slice and serve the creamy and caramel-infused Mexican Flan. Enjoy the classic dessert with its smooth texture and rich flavors, perfect for holiday feasting!
13. Enjoy exploring the diverse and delicious pies and cobblers from these countries as part of your holiday feasting!

SECTION V

COOKIES

AFRICA

COOKIES

Babazekhaya – Swaziland

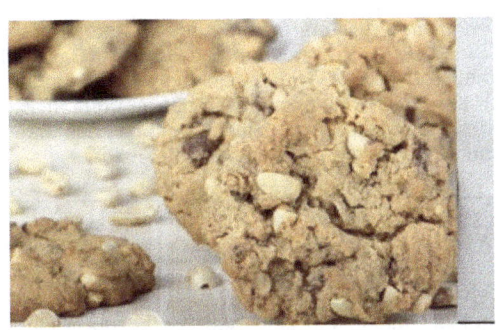

Swaziland is located in the heart of southern Africa with a rich and vibrant culture. Indulge with flavors and aromas that define Swazi desserts.

INGREDIENTS

- 1 cup ground peanuts
- 1 cup sugar
- 1 cup butter, softened
- 2 cups all-purpose flour

DIRECTIONS

1. Preheat your oven to (180°C).
2. Line a baking sheet with butter paper or parchment paper.
3. Cream the softened butter and sugar together in a mixing bowl until they are light and fluffy.
4. Add the ground peanuts and mix well.
5. Gradually add the flour to the mixture and mix until a dough forms.
6. Take a small part of the dough. Roll it into 1 and 1/2 inch thick ball.
7. Position the dough balls on the prepared baking sheet, ensuring they are spread out adequately.
8.
9. Bake the dough balls in the preheated oven for approximately 12-15 minutes, or until they turn a lovely golden brown color.
10. Once baked, take the cookies out of the oven and allow them to cool on the baking sheet for a few minutes.
11. Transfer the cookies from the baking sheet to a wire rack, giving them ample time to cool completely before serving

COOKIES

DaboKolo Cookies — Ethiopia

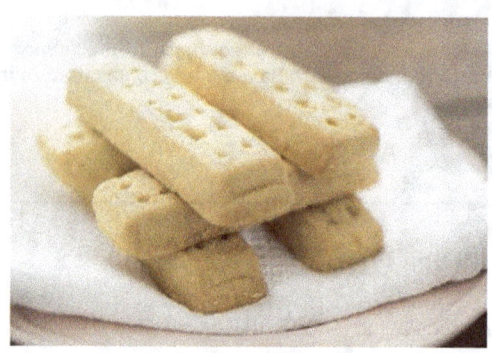

Ethiopia is renowned for its aromatic coffees, and its coffee-flavored desserts are a treat for the senses. Savor the delightful taste of Tiramisu with a uniquely Ethiopian twist, infused with the finest Ethiopian coffee beans. Don't miss out on the mouthwatering DaboKolo, small sweet pastries that will transport you to the bustling streets of Addis Ababa.

INGREDIENTS

- 2 cups all-purpose flour
- 1/2 cup unsalted butter, softened
- 1/2 cup sugar
- 1/2 teaspoon ground cardamom
- 1/2 teaspoon ground cinnamon
- Oil for frying

DIRECTIONS

1. Mix together sugar and softened butter until light and creamy.
2. Add the ground cardamom, ground cinnamon, and flour to th butter-sugar mixture. Mix until it becomes like a crumbly dough.
3. Knead the dough gently until it comes together and becomes smooth.
4. Pinch off small portions of the dough and roll them into small balls, about the size of marbles.
5. Heat oil in a deep frying pan or pot over medium heat.
6. Carefully drop the dough balls into the hot oil and fry them until they turn golden brown and crispy.
7. With the help of a slotted spoon, take out cookies on an absorbent paper towel to drain excess oil.
8. Let the cookies cool completely. They will become more crunchier as they cool before serving.

COOKIES

Kashata Cookies — Tanzania

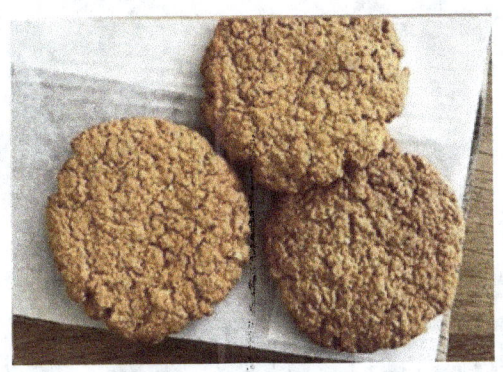

Tanzania is a true gem of East Africa. From the shores of the Indian Ocean to the majestic Serengeti plains, this country is a culinary delight. Indulge in the sumptuous Zanzibar Spice Cake. Let the sweet symphony of Tanzanian desserts tantalize your taste buds.

INGREDIENTS

- 2 cups desiccated coconut
- 1 cup granulated sugar
- 1 cup ground peanuts
- 1/2 cup water
- 1/2 teaspoon vanilla extract

DIRECTIONS

1. In a saucepan, combine the sugar and water. Cook on medium heat until the sugar dissolves completely. Stir continuously.
2. Add the desiccated coconut and ground peanuts to the saucepan.
3. Cook the mixture over low heat, stirring constantly, until it thickens and starts to pull away from the sides of the pan.
4. Turn off the heat. Add vanilla extract, and mix well.
5. Pour the mixture into a greased or lined baking dish and spread it out evenly.
6. Let the mixture cool and set completely. This can take a couple of hours.
7. Once set, cut the mixture into small bars or rounds.
8. Store the Kashata cookies in an airtight container until ready to serve.

ASIA

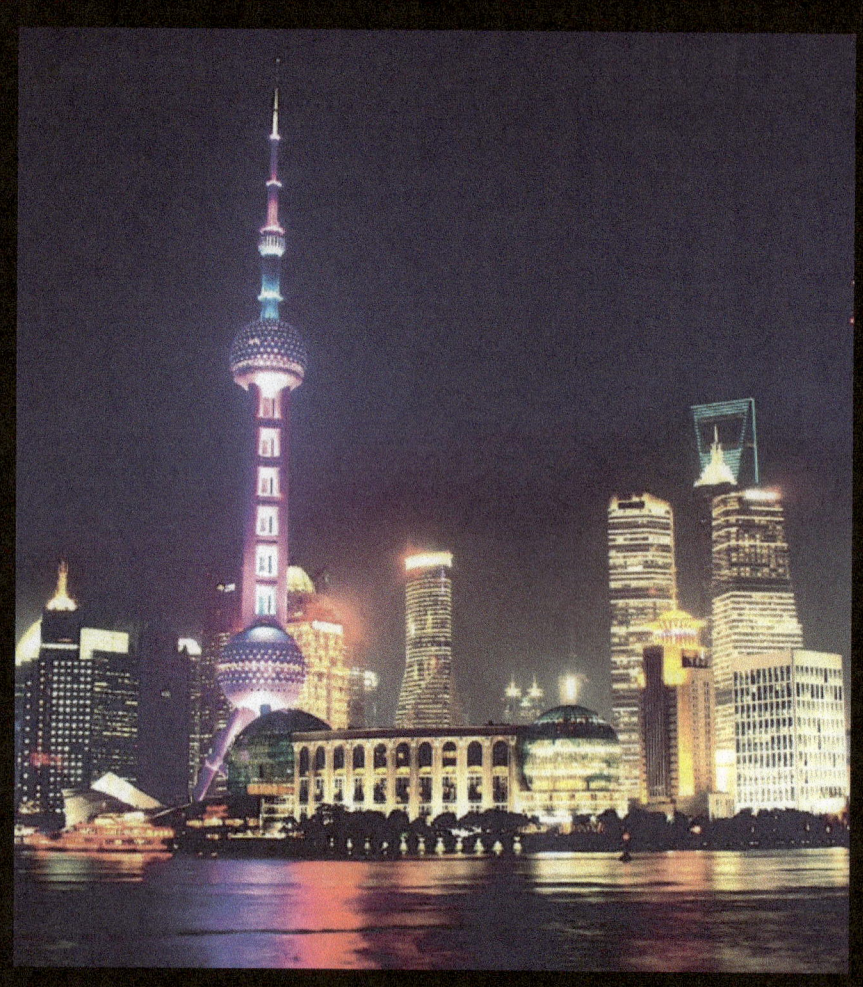

COOKIES

Matcha Green Tea Cookies — Japan

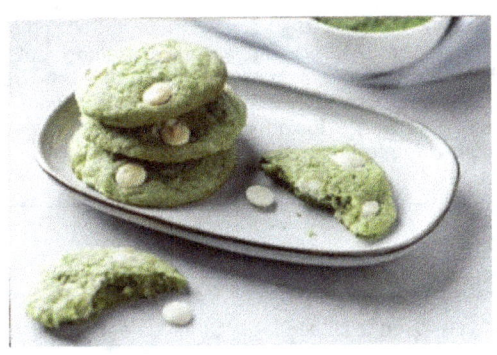

Japan land of the rising sun where desserts are a delicate balance of flavors, textures, and beautiful presentation. Experience the art of Wagashi, exquisite traditional confections made from sweetened bean paste, often shaped like delicate flowers or seasonal symbols. Indulge in the flavors of Matcha, a finely ground green tea powder used to create delightful desserts like Matcha Mochi or Matcha Parfaits.

INGREDIENTS

- 1 1/2 cups all-purpose flour
- 2 tablespoons matcha green tea powder
- 1/2 cup unsalted butter, softened
- 1/2 cup granulated sugar
- 1 egg yolk
- 1/2 teaspoon vanilla extract

DIRECTIONS

1. Preheat you oven to (180°C)
2. line a bakin sheet with butter paper or parchment paper.
3. In a mixing bowl, sift together the flour and matcha green tea powder.
4. In another bowl, mix butter and sugar until creamy, light and fluffy. Add egg yolk mixture and whisk again.
5. Add the flour mixture to the wet ingredients gradually. Mix until a soft and smooth dough forms.
6. Dust the working surface with flour.
7. Roll out dough. It must be 1/4 inch in thickness.
8. With the help of a glass or cookie cutter shape it into whatever you want
9. In a separate bowl, cream together the softened butter and sugar until light and fluffy.
10. Place the cut-out cookies on the prepared baking sheet, spacing them apart.
11. Bake in the preheated oven for 10-12 minutes or until the edges of the cookies are lightly golden.
12. Remove from the oven and let the cookies cool on the baking sheet for a few minutes.

COOKIES

KuehBangkit Cookies — Singapore

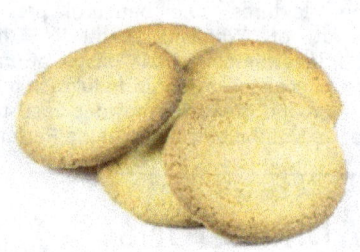

Singapore located in Asia is Known as a melting pot of cultures, this cosmopolitan destination offers desserts from various ethnic backgrounds. Explore the rich flavors of traditional desserts with a fusion of tastes and textures that will leave you craving for more.

INGREDIENTS

- 250g tapioca flour ⊠ 150g icing sugar
- 100g coconut milk
- 2 egg yolks
- Red food coloring (optional)
- Banana leaves (for presentation)

DIRECTIONS

1. Preheat your oven to 325°F (160°C) and line a baking sheet with parchment paper.
2. In a mixing bowl, combine the tapioca flour and icing sugar.
3. Add the coconut milk and egg yolks to the dry ingredients. Mix until a soft dough forms.
4. If desired, add a few drops of red food coloring to a small portion of the dough and mix well to create a contrasting color.
5. Dust the working surface with flour.
6. Roll out dough with 1/2 inch thickness.
7. Use cookie cutters or small-sized lids to cut out desired shapes from the dough.
8. Set cookies on the lined baking dish. Keep at a distance from each other.
9. Bake in the preheated oven for about 15-20 minutes
10. Discard cookies from the oven. Let them cool on baking sheets for a few minutes.
11. Then Cool cookies on a wire rack
12. For the presentation, you can place the cooled cookies on banana leaves or serve them in a decorative container.

COOKIES

Dasik Cookies — South Korea

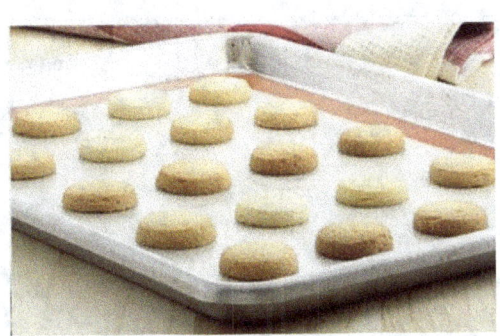

South Korea's desserts are as captivating as its pop culture. South Korea's desserts seamlessly blend tradition and contemporary making it a paradise for desserts.

INGREDIENTS

- 1 cup roasted grain powders (such as rice, sesame, and soybean)
- 1/4 cup honey or sugar
- Nuts or dried fruits for garnish (optional)

DIRECTIONS

1. Mix honey or powdered sugar and roasted grain powders. Mix until well combined.
2. You can also add chopped dry fruits or nuts to enhance the flavor.
3. Shape cookies with the help of molds or hands.
4. Cover the tray and rest for 1 hour to firm up.
5. Once firm, the cookies are ready to be enjoyed.

AUSTRALIA & OCEANIA

COOKIES

TeKawawong — Kiribati

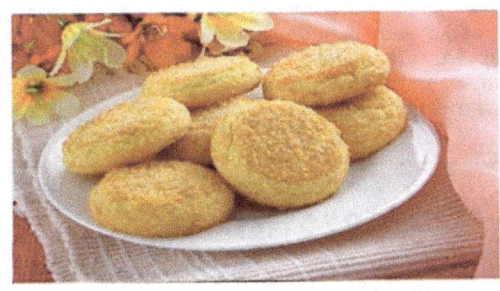

Kiribati, an island in the heart of the Pacific Ocean with breathtaking landscape. Kiribati desserts are a celebration of the bounties of the sea and the richness of local ingredients.

INGREDIENTS

- 2 cups grated coconut
- 1 cup sugar
- 1 1/2 cups all-purpose flour
- 1/2 cup butter, melted

DIRECTIONS

1. Preheat your oven to (180°C)
2. Line a baking sheet with butter paper or parchment paper.
3. In a mixing bowl, combine the grated coconut, sugar, flour, and melted butter. Mix well to form a dough.
4. Take small portions of the dough and roll them into small rounds.
5. Place the dough rounds on the prepared baking sheet, spacing them apart.
6. Bake in the preheated oven for about 15-20 minutes. Discard from the oven.
7. let the cookies cool on the baking sheet for a few minutes.
8. Then Cool on a wire rack.
9. Enjoy!

COOKIES

Tonya Coconut — Tonya

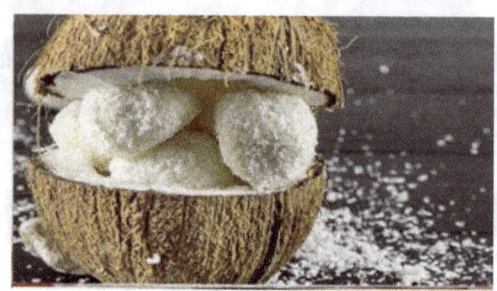

Tonya is located with beautiful beaches, and rich culture. Tonya's desserts are a delightful reflection of the island's tropical paradise. Indulge in the flavors of Tonya and experience a true taste of island sweetness.

INGREDIENTS

- 1 cup grated coconut
- 1 cup flour
- 1/2 cup sugar
- Pinch of salt
- 1/2 cup melted butter

DIRECTIONS

1. Preheat the oven to 350°F (175°C).
2. In a mixing bowl, combine 1 cup of grated coconut, 1 cup of flour, 1/2 cup of sugar, and a pinch of salt.
3. Add 1/2 cup of melted butter and mix well until the dough comes together.
4. Take small portions of the dough and shape them into cookies.
5. Place the cookies on a baking sheet and bake for about 15-20 minutes, or until they turn golden brown.
6. Allow the cookies to cool before serving.

COOKIES

Banana Bread Cookies — Palau

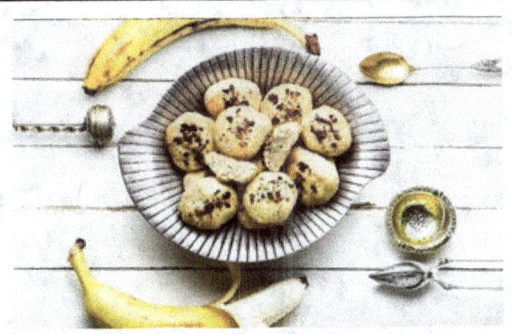

Palau is a paradise in the Pacific Ocean for both nature and dessert lovers. Enjoy its stunning landscapes and crystal-clear waters, along with its tasty desserts.

INGREDIENTS

- 2 ripe bananas
- 1/2 cup softened butter ⬚ 1/2 cup sugar
- 1/2 teaspoon cinnamon
- 1/2 teaspoon nutmeg
- 1 1/2 cups flour
- 1/2 teaspoon baking soda

DIRECTIONS

1. Preheat the oven to 375°F (190°C).
2. In a bowl, mash 2 ripe bananas until smooth.
3. Add 1/2 cup of softened butter, 1/2 cup of sugar, and 1/2 teaspoon each of cinnamon and nutmeg. Mix well.
4. Gradually add 1 1/2 cups of flour and 1/2 teaspoon of baking soda to the mixture. Stir until well combined.
5. With the help of an ice cream spoon, pour a drop of dough onto the baking tray.
6. Bake for approximately ten to twelve minutes.
7. Allow the cookies to cool before enjoying them.

EUROPE

COOKIES

French butter cookies — France

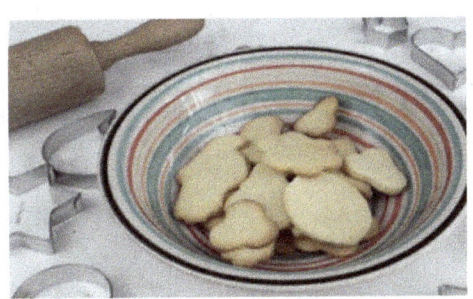

France is renowned for its mastery of patisserie, some of Europe & and the world's most exquisite sweets. France's desserts embody elegance and sophistication. Sablés are the classic French Butter Cookies. These delicate and buttery treats are loved for their melt-in-your-mouth texture.

INGREDIENTS

- 1 cup unsalted butter, softened
- 3/4 cup powdered sugar
- 2 egg yolks
- 2 teaspoons vanilla extract
- 2 1/2 cups all-purpose flour
- Pinch of sal
- Optional for decoration
- Additional powdered sugar

DIRECTIONS

1. Mix the sugar and softened butter until creamy and fluffy.
2. Add the egg yolks and vanilla extract to the bowl and mix until well combined.
3. Gradually add the flour and salt to the mixture, stirring until a smooth dough forms. Be careful not to overmix.
4. Shape the dough into a disk, wrap it in plastic wrap, and refrigerate for at least 1 hour or until firm
5. Preheat the oven to 175°C
6. Line a baking sheet with butter or parchment paper. Roll out the dough to 1/4 inch thickness.
7. Use cookie cutters to cut out desired shapes and transfer them to the prepared baking sheet. Leave some space between the cookies.
8. If desired, you can lightly sprinkle additional powdered sugar over the cookies for a decorative touch.
9. Bake in the preheated oven for approximately 10-12 minutes or until the edges of the cookies turn lightly golden.
10. Cool on a baking sheet for a few minutes.
11. Cool on a wire rack for 5 minutes. Then enjoy!
12. Once cooled, the French Butter Cookies are ready to be enjoyed!
13. These delightful French Butter Cookies are perfect for holiday gatherings, afternoon tea, or simply as a sweet treat to enjoy at home. Their rich buttery flavor and delicate texture make them a beloved addition to festive feasts. Bon appétit!

COOKIES

Croatian Kiflice — Croatia

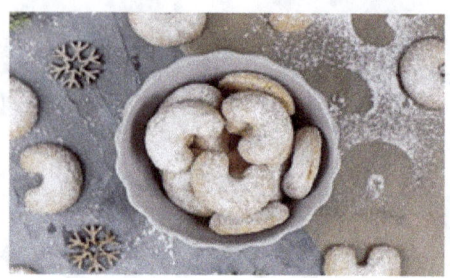

Croatiain located in southeastern Europe, boasts a rich culinary heritage and desserts. Kiflice - these crescent-shaped cookies filled with various sweet fillings reflect Croatia's culinary creativity.

INGREDIENTS

- 2 cups all-purpose flour
- 1/2 cup softened butter
- 1/2 cup plain yogurt
- 1/4 cup sugar
- Filling of choice (e.g., Nutella, jam, ground walnuts)
- Recipe Instructions:

DIRECTIONS

1. Preheat the oven to 350°F (175°C).
2. In a bowl, mix 2 cups of all-purpose flour, 1/2 cup of softened butter, 1/2 cup of plain yogurt, and 1/4 cup of sugar until a smooth dough forms.
3. Take the dough and divide it into small portions, then proceed to roll out each portion into a thin circle.
4. Cut each circle into wedges and add your desired sweet filling (e.g., Nutella, jam, or ground walnuts) on the wider end of each wedge.
5. Roll the dough from the wider end towards the pointed end to form a crescent shape.
6. Place the cookies on a baking sheet and bake for about 15-20 minutes, or until they become golden brown.
7. Let the cookies cool before serving.

COOKIES

Belarus Almond Nut Cookies — Belarus

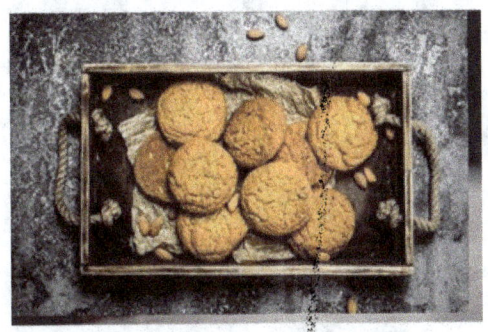

Belarus located in Eastern Europe, The Almond Nut Cookies are one of popular cookies, Crispy on the outside with a delightful almond flavor. these cookies capture the essence of Belarusian confectionery craftsmanship. Treat yourself to a taste of Belarus and discover a world of delightful surprises.

INGREDIENTS

- 1 cup ground almonds
- 1 cup sugar
- 2 egg whites
- Optional
- Whole almonds for decoration (optional

DIRECTIONS

1. Preheat the oven to 350°F (175°C).
2. In a mixing bowl, combine 1 cup of ground almonds, 1 cup of sugar, and 2 egg whites. Mix until well blended.
3. Using a spoon, place dollops of the dough onto a baking sheet that has been lined with parchment paper.
4. Optional: Place a whole almond on top of each cookie for decoration.
5. Bake for approximately 12-15 minutes or until the cookies turn golden brown.
6. Cool at room temperature before serving.

CARRIBBEAN

COOKIES

Jamaican Coconut Drops — Jamaica

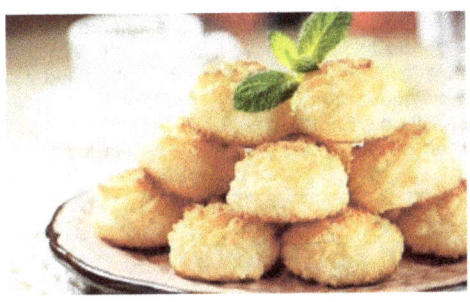

The Caribbean island of Jamaica not only captivates visitors with its vibrant culture and reggae rhythms but also with its irresistible desserts. The Coconut Drops is made with freshly grated coconut, spices, and a touch of sweetness, these chewy delights are a Jamaican favorite.

INGREDIENTS

- 2 cups grated coconut
- 1 cup sugar
- 1/4 cup water
- 1/2 teaspoon ground ginger
- 1/2 teaspoon ground cinnamon
- Pinch of salt

DIRECTIONS

1. In a saucepan, combine grated coconut, oil sugar, water, ground ginger, ground cinnamon, and a pinch of salt.
2. Cook the mixture over medium heat, stirring continuously, until the sugar dissolves and the mixture thickens.
3. Remove the saucepan from the heat and let the mixture cool slightly.
4. Drop a spoonful of the mixture onto a greased wax paper or baking sheet.
5. Let the coconut drops cool and harden before serving.

COOKIES

Guava Thumbprint Cookies — St. Kitts & Nevis

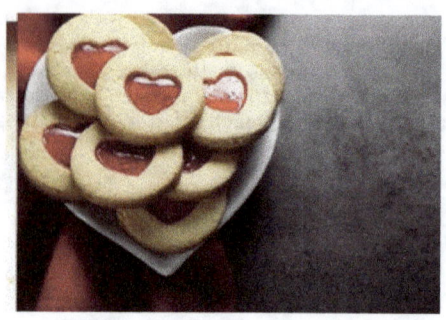

St. Kitts & Nevis in the Caribbean offers a unique dessert experience. Get ready to tantalize your taste buds with their Guava Thumbprint Cookies. These buttery delights, filled with the sweet tang of guava jam, perfectly capture the tropical essence of these islands. Explore the rich flavors of St. Kitts & Nevis and let their desserts leave an indelible mark on your palate

INGREDIENTS

- 1 cup unsalted butter, softened
- 1/2 cup granulated sugar
- 2 cups all-purpose flour
- A pinch of salt
- Guava jam

DIRECTIONS

1. Preheat your oven to 350°F (175°C).
2. In a mixing bowl, cream together the softened butter and granulated sugar until the mixture becomes light and fluffy.
3. Mix salt and flour until a smooth dough forms.
4. Take small parts of the dough in your hands
5. Roll them into small-sized balls.
6. Place these dough balls onto a baking sheet, making sure to leave enough space between each cookie.
7. Create an indentation in the center of each cookie using either your thumb or the back of a spoon.
8. Fill each indentation with a dollop of guava jam, making sure not to overfill.
9. Place the baking sheet in the preheated oven and bake for approximately 13-15 minutes depending on your oven. Check after 13 minutes for best results.
10. Once baked, remove the cookies from the oven and allow them to cool completely on a wire rack before enjoying their deliciousness

COOKIES

Bermuda Rum Delights — Bermuda

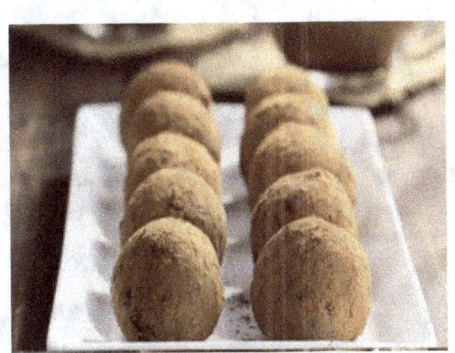

Bermuda is located in the North Atlantic Ocean with beautiful pink-sandy beaches and vibrant culture but also for its delightful Rum Swizzle Cookies. Mixed with the flavors of rum and citrus, these cookies reflect the island's spirit of relaxation and indulgence. Treat yourself to a taste of Bermuda and let the flavors transport you to a place of pure tropical bliss.

INGREDIENTS

- 1/2 cup softened butter
- 1 cup brown sugar
- 3 tablespoons dark rum
- 1 teaspoon freshly grated lime zest
- 1 teaspoon freshly grated lemon zest
- 2 cups all-purpose flour
- Pinch of salt

DIRECTIONS

1. Preheat the oven to 350°F (175°C).
2. In a mixing bowl, cream together the softened butter and brown sugar until creamy and well combined.
3. Add the dark rum, lime zest, and lemon zest to the mixture. Mix thoroughly.
4. Gradually add the all-purpose flour and a pinch of salt to the mixture, stirring until a dough forms.
5. Create small round-shaped balls from the dough and set them on a cookie sheet.
6. Gently press down on each ball with the back of a spoon to flatten them slightly.
7. Bake for 10-12 minutes.
8. Cool cookies on a wire rack for a few minutes before serving.

South America & Latin America

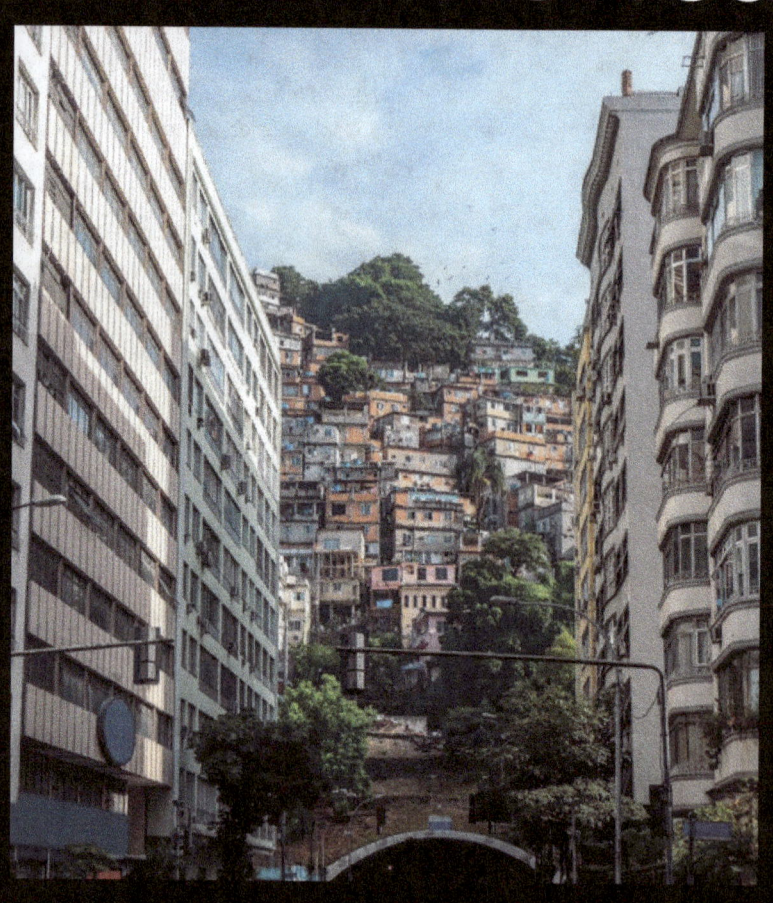

COOKIES

Ecuadorian Dulce Delights — Ecuador

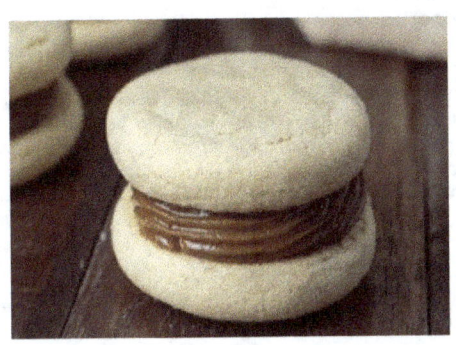

Ecuador is Located in South America with a beautiful landscapes and rich culinary heritage. Alfajores is a popular dessertsandwich cookies filled with dulce de leche, a sweet celebration of Ecuador's culinary creativity and rich, creamy flavors.

INGREDIENTS

- 1 cup softened butter
- 1/2 cup powdered sugar
- 2 cups all-purpose flour
- 1/4 teaspoon baking powder
- Dulce de leche

DIRECTIONS

1. Preheat the oven to 350°F (175°C).
2. Mix sugar and butter in a wide bowl until creamy and fluffy.
3. Add the all-purpose flour and baking powder to the mixture. Mix until the dough comes together.
4. Dust the working surface with flour, and roll out the dough on it.
5. Keep dough 1/4 inch in thickness.
6. Use a cookie cutter to cut out small rounds or desired shapes.
7. Place the cookies on a baking sheet and bake for about 10-12 minutes or until lightly golden.
8. Allow the cookies to cool completely.
9. Spread a layer of dulce de leche on the bottom side of one cookie and sandwich it with another cookie.
10. Repeat with the remaining cookies.
11. Optional: Dust the tops of the dulce delights with powdered sugar before serving.

COOKIES

Vibrant Venezuelan Crumbles — Venezuela

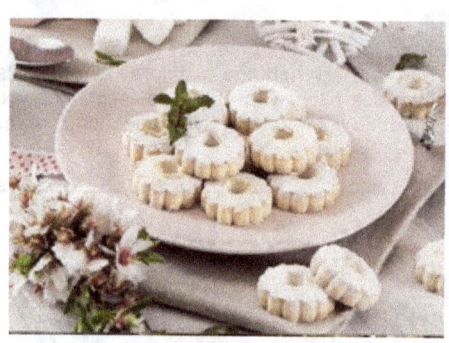

Located on the northern coast of South America, Venezuela has a vibrant dessert culture The beloved Polvorosas, crumbly and buttery cookies coated in powdered sugar, hold a special place in Venezuelan hearts. With their delicate texture and melt-in-yourmouth goodness, these cookies capture the essence of Venezuela's passion for creating desserts that bring joy to every bite.

INGREDIENTS

- 1 cup softened butter
- 1/2 cup powdered sugar
- 1/2 cup powdered sugar 2 cups all-purpose flour Pinch of salt

DIRECTIONS

1. Preheat the oven to 350°F (175°C).
2. Mix butter and sugar in a wide bowl until creamy and fluffy
3. Add flour and 1/4 teaspoon of salt to the mixture. Mix until a smooth and cohesive dough forms.
4. Make small balls out of dough.
5. Set them on a baking tray.
6. Bake for 11- 15 minutes. Check after 12 minutes. Temperature may vary depending on your oven.
7. Discard cookies from the oven.
8. Cool them on a wire rack for 5 minutes. Then roll into icing sugar or powdered sugar.
9. Cool them completely before serving

COOKIES

Panamanian Coconut Delights — Panama

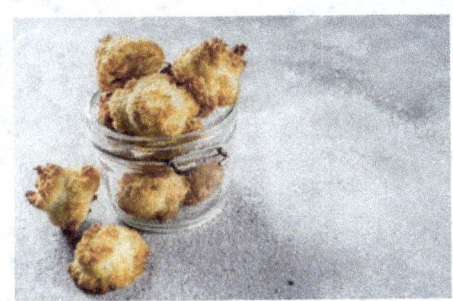

Located in Central America, Panama culinary delights include Cocadas. These chewy and sweet cookies, made with coconut and condensed milk, offer a taste of tropical paradise with each bite. Be transported to the sunny beaches of Panama as you savor the flavors of these delightful treats.

INGREDIENTS

- 2 cups shredded coconut
- 1 cup sweetened condensed milk

DIRECTIONS

1. Preheat the oven to 350°F (175°C).
2. In a mixing bowl, combine the shredded coconut and sweetened condensed milk. Mix well.
3. Put a spoonful of the mixture onto a baking sheet covered with parchment paper.
4. Bake for about 15-20 minutes or until the edges of the cookies become golden brown.
5. Take the cookies out of the oven and let them cool on the baking sheet for a little while.
6. Move the cookies onto a wire rack and let them cool completely.
7. Serve the coconut delights once they have cooled down.

NORTH AMERICA

COOKIES

US Mountain Bliss Cookies — Colorado

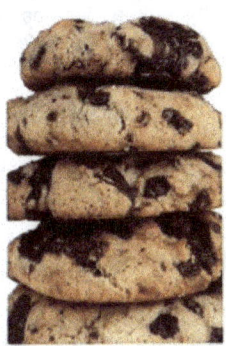

Known for its stunning Rocky Mountains and outdoor adventures, Colorado also has some delectable dessertsthat are as diverse and vibrant as its landscapes. Indulge in these delightful treats and experience the sweet side of the Centennial State.

INGREDIENTS

- 1 cup unsalted butter, softened
- 1 cup granulated sugar
- 1 cup packed brown sugar
- 2 large eggs
- 1 teaspoon vanilla extract
- 3 cups all-purpose flour
- 1 teaspoon baking powder
- 1/2 teaspoon salt
- 2 cups semisweet chocolate chips

DIRECTIONS

1. Preheat the oven to 375°F (190°C).
2. Sift all-purpose flour, baking powder, and salt.
3. Mix butter and sugar in a wide bowl until creamy and fluffy
4. Whisk in eggs and vanilla extract and beat again.
5. Add dry ingredients to the wet ingredients gradually. Mix well with a spatula with light hands.
6. Stir in the semisweet chocolate chips.
7. Drop a rounded spoonful of dough onto a baking sheet, spacing them about 2 inches apart.
8. Bake for approximately 9-11 minutes, or until the edges are lightly golden.
9. Cool cookies on the baking tray.
10. Then Cool on a wire rack. This step makes them more crispier.

COOKIES

Maple Pecan Delights of Montreal — Montreal, Canada

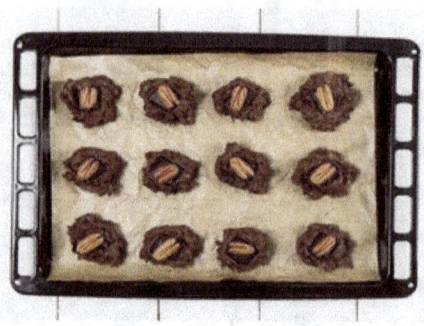

Imagine the smell of freshly baked pastries and desserts through the air. This Canadian city is a haven for dessert lovers, offering a range of delectable treats. Sink your teeth into Maple Pecan Cookies, a delightful combination of sweet maple syrup and crunchy pecans that pays homage to Canada's iconic maple syrup industry. Discover the sweet side of Montreal and let its desserts captivate your taste buds.

INGREDIENTS

- 1 cup unsalted butter, softened
- 1 cup packed brown sugar
- 1/2 cup granulated sugar
- 2 large eggs
- 1 teaspoon vanilla extract
- 2 cups all-purpose flour ▢ 1 teaspoon baking soda
- 1/2 teaspoon salt
- 1 cup chopped pecans
- 1/2 cup pure maple syrup

DIRECTIONS

1. Preheat the oven to 350°F (175°C).
2. Sift all-purpose flour, baking powder, and salt
3. Mix butter and sugar in a wide bowl until creamy and fluffy
4. Whisk in eggs and vanilla extract and beat again
5. Add dry ingredients to the wet ingredients gradually.
6. Mix well with a spatula with light hands
7. Stir in the chopped pecans.
8. Drizzle the pure maple syrup over the dough and gently fold it in until evenly distributed.
9. Drop rounded spoonful of dough onto a baking sheet, spacing them about 2 inches apart.
10. Bake for approximately 9-11 minutes, or until the edges are lightly golden.
11. Cool cookies on the baking tray

COOKIES

Coconut Lime Bites — TULUM, Mexico

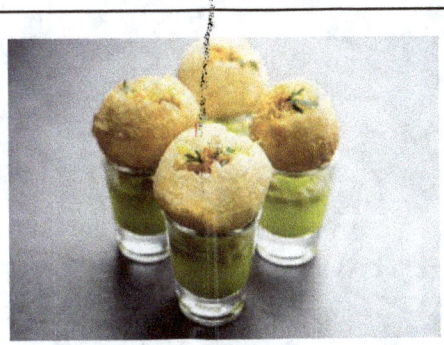

Located on the Caribbean coastline of Mexico's Quintana Roo region, Tulum not only offers breathtaking beaches but also a vibrant dessert culture. Embrace the tropical flavors of the area with Coconut Lime Cookies. These delightful treats combine the tropical sweetness of coconut with the zesty tang of lime, perfectly capturing the essence of Tulum's laid-back paradise. Treat yourself to these cookies and let the flavors transport you to the sundrenched shores of Quintana Roo.

INGREDIENTS

- 1 cup unsalted butter, softened
- 1 cup granulated sugar
- 1 large egg
- 1 teaspoon vanilla extract
- 2 cups all-purpose flour
- 1 teaspoon baking powder
- 1/2 teaspoon salt
- Zest of 2 limes
- 1/2 cup shredded coconut

DIRECTIONS

1. Preheat the oven to 350°F (175°C).
2. Sift all-purpose flour, baking powder, and salt.
3. Mix butter and sugar until creamy and light.
4. Add vanilla extract and eggs and whisk well with a beater at medium speed.
5. Add dry ingredients to the wet ingredients gradually. Mix well with a spatula with light hands
6. Add shredded coconut and lime zest.
7. Drop a rounded spoonful of dough onto a baking sheet, spacing them about 2 inches apart.
8. Bake for ten to twelve minutes.
9. Enjoy baking and savoring these delicious cookies from around the world.

SECTION VI

ICE CREAM

AFRICA

ICE CREAM

Sahrawi Tea Ice Cream — Western Sahara

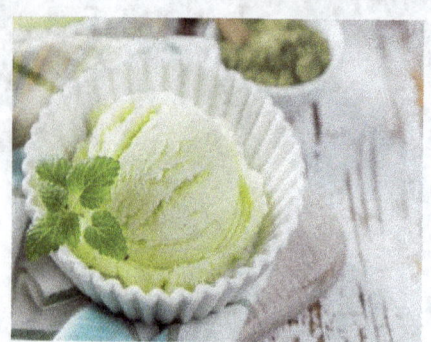

Western Sahara is located In desert region of Africa. Sahrawi Tea Ice Cream combines the flavors of green tea and sweetened condensed milk, creating a unique and delightful frozen treat

INGREDIENTS

- 1 ½ cup heavy cream
- 1 ½ cup whole milk
- 3 tbsp Thai tea mix
- 6 egg yolks
- ¼ cup condensed milk
- ¼ cup granulated sugar
- 1 tsp vanilla extract
- ¼ tsp salt
- 1 oz dark chocolate optional
- 1 tsp coconut oil optional

DIRECTIONS

1. Brew a strong pot of Sahrawi tea, using loose green tea leaves and plenty of sugar.
2. Let the tea cool to room temperature.
3. Mix the cooled tea with sweetened condensed milk until well combined.
4. Pour the mixture into an ice cream maker and churn until the mixture turns creamy.
5. Once churned, transfer the ice cream to a container and freeze for a few hours until firm.
6. Serve the Sahrawi Tea Ice Cream in bowls or cones and enjoy the unique flavors of the Western Sahara.

ICE CREAM

Pineapple and Ginger Ice Cream — Zambia

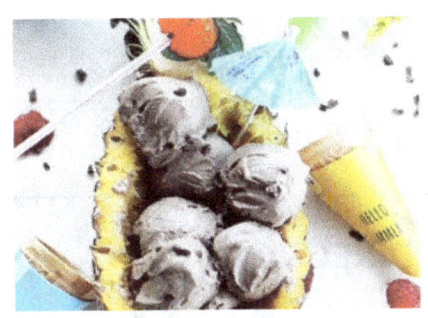

Zambia's tropical climate and abundant fruits inspire "Pineapple and Ginger Ice Cream." This vibrant dessert blends the sweetness of ripe pineapples with a hint of zesty ginger, resulting in a tropical paradise in every spoon.

INGREDIENTS

- cheesecloth
- gingerroot 40 g
- fresh cilantro 2 1/2 tbsp
- vanilla ice cream 4 scoops
- pineapple 2/3

DIRECTIONS

1. Peel and core a ripe pineapple, then chop it into small chunks.
2. In a blender, combine the pineapple chunks, grated fresh ginger, and a squeeze of lime juice.
3. Blend until smooth.
4. In a separate bowl, whisk together heavy cream, sugar, and vanilla extract until well combined.
5. Add the pineapple-ginger mixture to the cream mixture and stir gently.
6. Pour mixture into ice cream maker and churn until mixture thickens and gets creamy.
7. Transfer the ice cream to a container and freeze for a few hours until it hardens.
8. Serve the Pineapple and Ginger Ice Cream in scoops and savor the tropical flavors of Zambia.

ICE CREAM

Masala Chai Ice Cream — Kenya

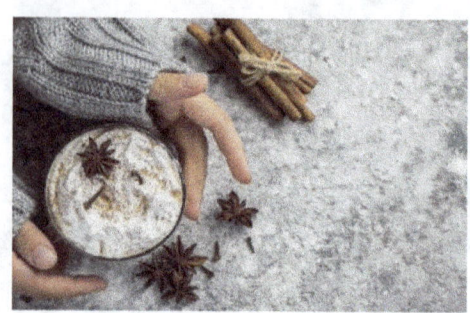

Embracing the aromatic and warm spices of the region, "Masala Chai Ice Cream" pays homage to Kenya's love for tea. The blend of black tea, cardamom, cinnamon, and ginger creates a delightful frozen rendition of the traditional Masala Chai.

INGREDIENTS

- 250 Ml Milk
- 100 gram Cream
- 100 gram Sugar
- 3 Egg yolks
- 3 tsp Masala tea powder
- 4 tbsp Tea (concentrated)

DIRECTIONS

1. In a saucepan, combine milk, heavy cream, and a mixture of black tea leaves, crushed cardamom pods, cinnamon sticks, and grated ginger. Simmer this mixture on medium heat.
2. Remove from heat, cover the saucepan, and let the flavors infuse for about 15 minutes.
3. To discard tea leaves and spices, strain this mixture.
4. In another bowl beat egg yolks and sugar until creamy and pale in color.
5. Slowly pour the warm milk mixture into the egg yolk mixture, whisking continuously.
6. Return the mixture to the saucepan.
7. Cook the mixture over low heat.
8. Stir constantly during the cooking process.
9. Wait until the mixture thickens.
10. Observe the mixture coating the back of a spoon.
11. Remove the saucepan from the heat source.
12. Allow the mixture to cool completely.
13. Pour the cooled mixture into an ice cream maker and churn until smooth and creamy.
14. Transfer the ice cream to a container and freeze for a few hours until set.
15. Serve the Masala Chai Ice Cream in bowls or cones, capturing the delightful flavors of Kenya.

ASIA

ICE CREAM

Mango Kulfi — India

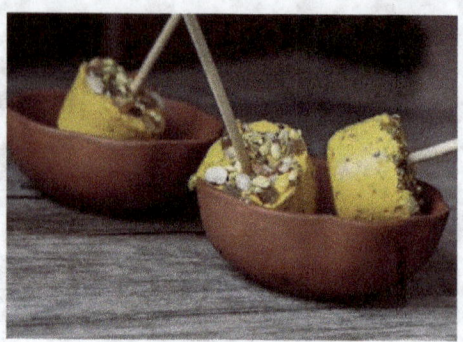

India's king of fruits takes the spotlight with "Mango Kulfi," a creamy and indulgent ice cream that captures the rich and luscious flavors of ripe mangoes, accented with cardamom and saffron.

INGREDIENTS

- 2 ripe mangoes, peeled and chopped
- (removing any fibrous parts)
- 1 can (14 ounces) condensed milk
- 1/2 teaspoon cardamom powder
- a few saffron threads
- 2 cups milk
- Chopped pistachios (for garnish

DIRECTIONS

1. Peel and chop ripe mangoes, removing any fibrous parts.
2. In a blender, blend the mango chunks, condensed milk, cardamom powder, and saffron threads until smooth.
3. In a saucepan, heat the milk until it starts to boil.
4. Add the mango mixture to the hot milk and simmer for a few minutes, stirring continuously.
5. Turn off the heat. Cool down the mixture at room temperature.
6. Pour the cooled mixture into molds or small bowls and freeze for at least 6 hours or until firm.
7. Serve the Mango Kulfi garnished with chopped pistachios, enjoying the rich and creamy Indian delight.

ICE CREAM

Almond and Rose Ice Cream— Nepal

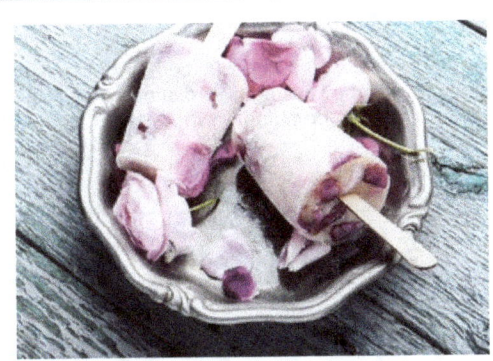

Offers a delicate and fragrant experience with a blend of blanched almonds, rose water, and cardamom. This frozen delight is a tribute to the country's refined taste for subtle flavors.

INGREDIENTS

- 1 cup blanched almonds
- 1 cup milk
- 2 cups heavy cream
- 1 tablespoon rose water
- 1/2 teaspoon cardamom powder
- 1 can (14 ounces) condensed milk

DIRECTIONS

1. In a blender, blend blanched almonds, milk, heavy cream, rose water, and a pinch of cardamom powder until smooth.
2. Add condensed milk and blend again until well combined.
3. Pour the mixture into an ice cream maker and continue churning until it thickens to the desired consistency.
4. Transfer the ice cream to a container and freeze for a few hours until it reaches the desired consistency.
5. Serve the Almond and Rose Ice Cream in bowls or cones, reveling in the delicate flavors of Nepal.

ICE CREAM

Durian Ice Cream — Indonesia

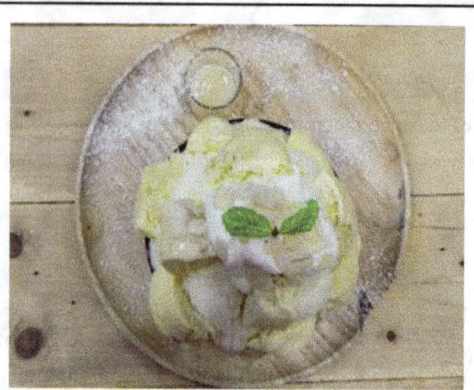

From the tropical paradise of Indonesia comes "Durian Ice Cream," a unique treat showcasing the distinct and robust flavors of ripe durian fruit, combined with creamy coconut milk.

INGREDIENTS

- 2 cups ripe durian flesh, seeds and outer skin removed
- 1 cup coconut milk
- 1/2 cup sweetened condensed milk
- Juice of 1 lime

DIRECTIONS

1. Cut open a ripe durian and remove the flesh, discarding the seeds and outer skin.
2. In a blender, blend the durian flesh, coconut milk, sweetened condensed milk, and a squeeze of lime juice until smooth.
3. Pour the mixture into an ice cream maker and churn until it thickens.
4. Transfer the ice cream to a container and freeze for several hours until it hardens.
5. Serve the Durian Ice Cream in scoops, embracing the distinct tropical taste of Indonesia.

AUSTRALIA & OCEANIA

ICE CREAM

Coconut Pandanus Ice Cream— Marshall Islands

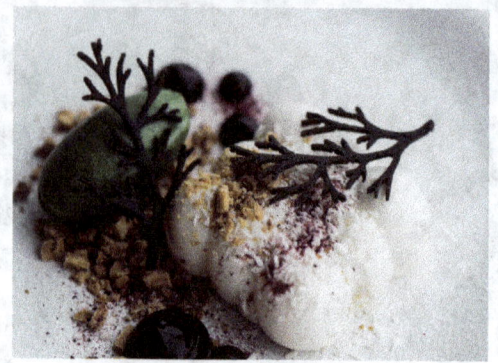

Coconut Pandanus Ice Cream" from the Marshall Islands celebrates the abundance of coconuts in the region. Enhanced with pandanus extract for a delightful twist, this frozen delight offers a taste of paradise. Coconut Pandanus Ice Cream

INGREDIENTS

- 2 cups coconut milk
- 1 cup heavy cream
- 1/2 cup sugar
- 1 tablespoon pandanus extract (optional)
- 4 large egg yolks

DIRECTIONS

1. Cut open a ripe durian and remove the flesh, discarding the seeds and outer skin.
2. In a blender, blend the durian flesh, coconut milk, sweetened condensed milk, and a squeeze of lime juice until smooth.
3. Pour the mixture into an ice cream maker and churn until it thickens.
4. Transfer the ice cream to a container and freeze for several hours until it hardens.
5. Serve the Durian Ice Cream in scoops, embracing the distinct tropical taste of Indonesia.

ICE CREAM

Coconut Lime Surprise Ice Cream - Niue

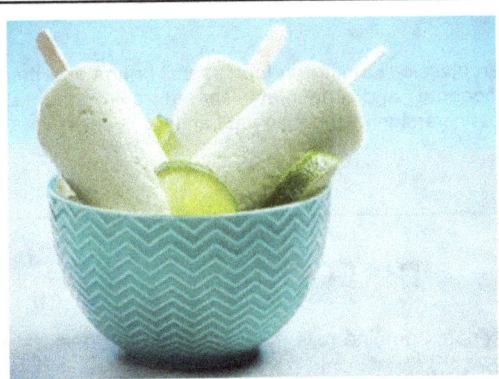

The South Pacific island nation of Niue comes "Coconut Lime Surprise Ice Cream," blending the tropical flavors of coconut and zesty lime for a refreshing and unique treat.

INGREDIENTS

- 1 cup coconut milk ⊠ 1 cup heavy cream
- 1/2 cup sweetened condensed milk
- Zest of 2 lime
- Juice of 1 lime ⊠ 1/4 cup shredded coconut (toasted)

DIRECTIONS

1. In a bowl, whisk together the coconut milk, heavy cream, sweetened condensed milk, lime zest, and lime juice.
2. Pour the mixture into an ice cream maker and churn until the mixture thickens. Follow the manufacturer's instructions strictly.
3. During the last few minutes of churning, add the toasted shredded coconut.
4. Transfer the ice cream to an airtight container and freeze for a few hours until firm.
5. Serve in cones or chilled bowls and enjoy the tropical flavors of Niue.

ICE CREAM

Lamington Ice Cream— Australia

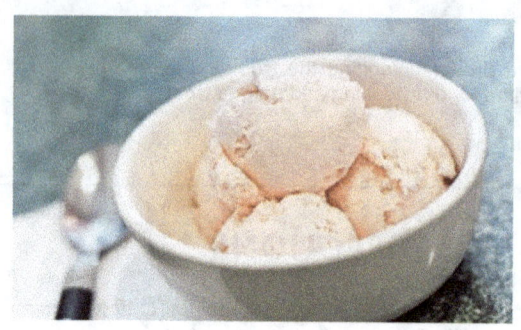

The Australian classic "Lamington Ice Cream" brings together desiccated coconut and chocolate sponge cake chunks, creating a frozen version of the beloved Lamington cake.

INGREDIENTS

- 2 cups milk
- 1 cup heavy cream
- 1/2 cup desiccated coconut
- 1/2 cup granulated sugar
- 4 large egg yolks
- 1 1/2 cups chocolate sponge cake, cut into small chunks

DIRECTIONS

1. In a saucepan, combine milk, heavy cream, and desiccated coconut.
2. Simmer the mixture on medium flame.
3. Remove from heat, cover the saucepan, and let it infuse for about 15 minutes.
4. Strain the mixture to remove the coconut.
5. In another bowl, beat egg yolks and sugar until the mixture turns creamy.
6. Slowly pour the warm milk mixture into the egg yolk mixture, whisking continuously.
7. Cook on low flame and stir continuously until the mixture thickens.
8. Turn off the heat. Cool this mixture at room temperature.
9. Once cooled, add chunks of chocolate sponge cake and mix gently.
10. Pour the mixture into an ice cream maker and churn it until it gets thick and creamy.
11. Transfer the ice cream to a container and freeze until set.
12. Serve the Lamington Ice Cream in scoops, savoring the Australian classic in frozen form.

EUROPE

ICE CREAM

Belgian Chocolate Ice Cream — Belgium

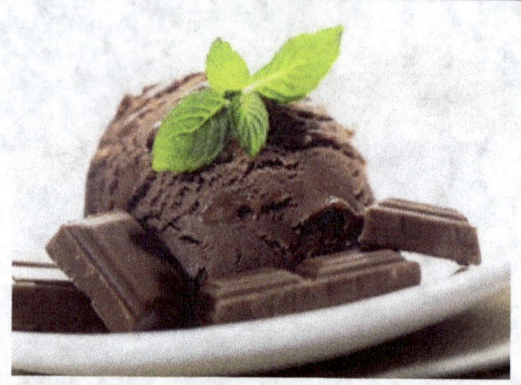

Europe is a continent with diverse cultures and cuisines. European-style ice cream is known for its creamy texture and rich flavors. For a classic European holiday treat, we have "Belgian Chocolate Ice Cream.

INGREDIENTS

- 2 cups heavy cream
- 1 cup whole milk
- 3/4 cup granulated sugar
- 1/2 cup unsweetened cocoa powder
- 4 large egg yolks
- 4 ounces Belgian chocolate (chopped)
- 1 teaspoon vanilla extract

DIRECTIONS

1. In a saucepan, heat the milk, cocoa powder, and heavy cream on medium heat.
2. Cook until it simmers while stirring continuously.
3. In another bowl, beat the egg yolks until custard-like consistency and are pale yellow in color
4. Slowly pour the hot cream mixture into the egg yolks, stirring constantly.
5. Then cook this mixture on the stove on low flame.
6. Stir until the mixture thickens.
7. Add the chopped Belgian chocolate. Mix until the c. Stir until you get a smooth mixture.
8. Lastly, add vanilla extract.
9. Cool this mixture and refrigerate for overnight or a minimum of 5 hours.
10. Churn the chilled mixture in an ice cream maker. Follow the manufacturer's instructions.
11. Transfer to a container, cover, and freeze until firm.
12. Serve in decadent scoops and indulge in the luscious flavors of European chocolate.

ICE CREAM

Sahlep Ice Cream — Turkey

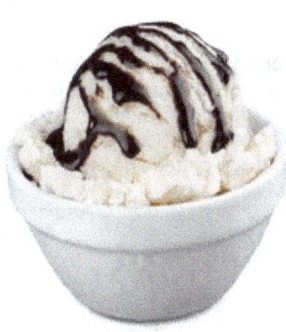

INGREDIENTS

- 2 cups milk
- 1 cup heavy cream
- 1/2 cup granulated suga
- 3 tablespoons sahlep powder
- 1 teaspoon rosewater (optional)
- Chopped pistachios for garnish

Turkey, a transcontinental country, boasts a rich culinary heritage that combines Middle Eastern, Central Asian, and Mediterranean influences.Sahlep Ice Cream represents Turkey's unique culinary heritage with its special ingredient called sahlep, derived from wild orchids. This ice cream is a delightful blend of exotic flavors.

DIRECTIONS

1. In a saucepan, heat the milk, heavy cream, and sugar over medium heat, stirring until the sugar dissolves.
2. Gradually whisk in the schlep powder, stirring constantly to avoid lumps. Continue cooking the mixture until it thickens to a custard-like consistency. Cool it at room temperature.
3. Add some rose water to enhance the flavor of this tempting ice cream.
4. Pour mixture into ice cream maker and churn as the manufacturer instructed. Follow their guidelines for the best results
5. Once churned, transfer the ice cream to a lidded container and freeze for a few hours until it's ready to serve.
6. Sprinkle chopped pistachios on top for an authentic Turkish touch and enjoy the creamy delights of Sahlep Ice Cream.

ICE CREAM

Zapekanka Ice Cream — Belarus

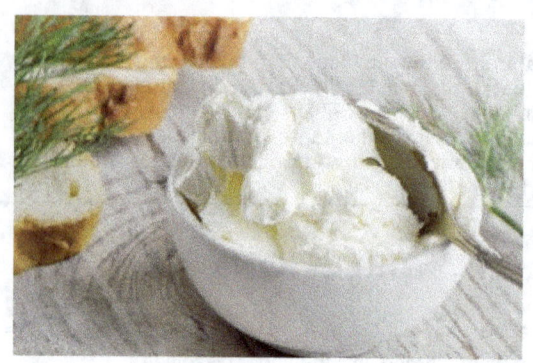

"Zapekanka Ice Cream" brings the charm of Belarusian cuisine with a creamy blend of cottage cheese, mixed dried fruits, and crushed biscuits for a delightful frozen experience. For a Belarusian holiday treat, we have "Zapekanka Ice Cream," inspired by the popular cottage cheese dessert.

INGREDIENTS

- 2 cups cottage cheese
- 1 cup heavy cream
- 1/2 cup powdered sugar
- 1 teaspoon vanilla extract
- 1/2 cup mixed dried fruits (raisins, apricots, cranberries)
- 1/4 cup crushed biscuits or cookies

DIRECTIONS

1. In a food processor, blend the cottage cheese, heavy cream, powdered sugar, and vanilla extract until smooth and creamy.
2. Fold in the mixed dried fruits and crushed biscuits, distributing them evenly.
3. Pour the mixture into an ice cream maker and churn until the mixture thickens.
4. Follow the manufacturer's instructions strictly.
5. Pour the ice cream mixture into an airtight container. Freeze until it reaches the desired consistency.
6. Serve in bowls or cones, and savor the unique taste of Belarusian Zapekanka Ice Cream.

ICE CREAM

Tiramisu Gelato— Italy

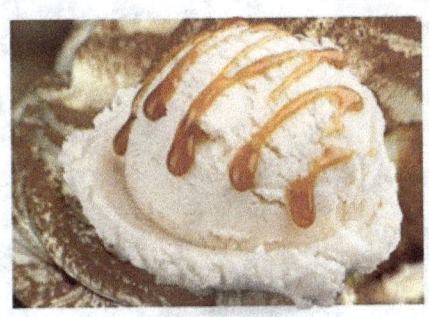

Italy's renowned gelato takes center stage with "Tiramisu Gelato," featuring the heavenly combination of coffee, mascarpone cheese, and ladyfingers in a velvety frozen form.

INGREDIENTS

- 1 cup whole milk
- 1 cup heavy cream
- 1/2 cup granulated sugar
- 4 large egg yolks
- 2 tablespoons instant coffee powder(mix in 4 tabspoon of hot water) (dissolved in 1/4 cup hot water)
- 1/4 cup coffee liqueur (optional)
- 1/2 cup mascarpone cheese
- 1/2 cup ladyfingers (crumbled)

DIRECTIONS

1. In a saucepan, heat the whole milk, heavy cream, and half of the granulated sugar over medium heat, stirring until it simmers.
2. In another bowl, beat the egg yolks with the remaining sugar until thick and pale in color.
3. Slowly pour the hot milk mixture into the egg yolks, stirring until the mixture thickens.
4. Cool this mixture at room temperature.
5. Pour the ice cream mixture into an air-tight container and freeze until it reaches the perfect gelato consistency.
6. Serve the Tiramisu Gelato in elegant bowls or waffle cones, and enjoy the divine flavors reminiscent of the famous Italian dessert, Tiramisu.

CARIBBEAN

ICE CREAM

Coconut Rum Ice Cream

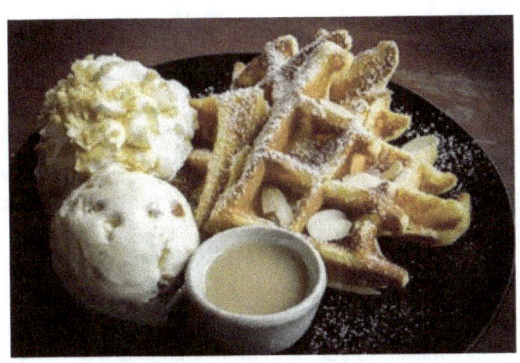

Italy's renowned gelato takes center stage with "Tiramisu Gelato," featuring the heavenly combination of coffee, mascarpone cheese, and ladyfingers in a velvety frozen form.

INGREDIENTS

- 2 cups coconut milk
- 1 cup heavy cream
- 1 cup sugar
- 4 egg yolks
- 1 teaspoon vanilla extract

DIRECTIONS

1. In a saucepan, heat the heavy cream and coconut milk on medium flame until it simmers.
2. In another bowl, beat egg yolks and sugar well.
3. Slowly pour the heated coconut milk and cream mixture into the egg yolks. Stir continuously to avoid any lumps in the mixture.
4. Cook this mixture on the stove on low flame.
5. Stir continuously until the mixture thickens.
6. Add run and vanilla extract
7. Cool this mixture and pour it into the ice cream maker .Churn by following the manufacturer's instructions.
8. Once churned, transfer the ice cream to a container and freeze for at least 4 hours or until firm.
9. Serve the Coconut Rum Ice Cream in bowls or cones, and enjoy the tropical flavors of the Caribbean!

ICE CREAM

Key Lime Pie Ice Cream — Cayman Islands

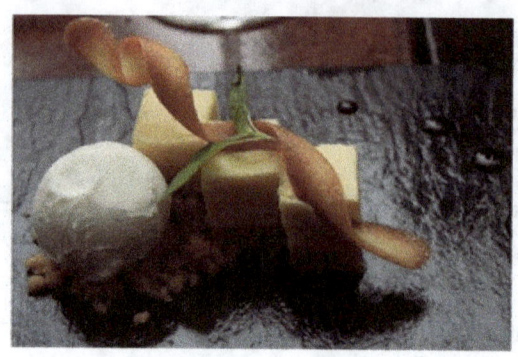

"Key Lime Pie Ice Cream" embodies the flavors of the Cayman Islands, combining tangy key limes with graham cracker crumbs for a tropical twist on the classic American dessert. A delightful ice cream recipe from this destination is the Key Lime Pie Ice Cream.

INGREDIENTS

- 2 cups heavy cream
- 1 cup whole milk
- 3/4 cup granulated sugar
- 4 large egg yolks
- 1/3 cup key lime juice
- 1 tablespoon key lime zest
- 1 cup graham cracker crumbs

DIRECTIONS

1. In a saucepan, heat the sugar, milk, and heavy cream. Heavy cream, milk, and sugar on medium flame.
2. Cook until it simmers. Stir continuously.
3. In another bowl, beat the egg yolks until the mixture turns into a custard-like thick consistency.
4. Slowly pour the hot cream mixture into the egg yolks, whisking constantly.
5. Cook the mixture on low flame until it thickens. Add lime juice and zest.
6. Cool this mixture at room temperature.
7. Then churn by following the manufacturer's instructions
8. In the last few seconds of churning, add graham crackers to the ice cream mixture.
9. Transfer the Key Lime Pie Ice Cream to a container and freeze for a few hours until firm.
10. Serve scoops of the ice cream in bowls or cones, and savor the tangy and refreshing taste of the Cayman Islands

ICE CREAM

Banana Flambé Ice Cream — Guadeloupe

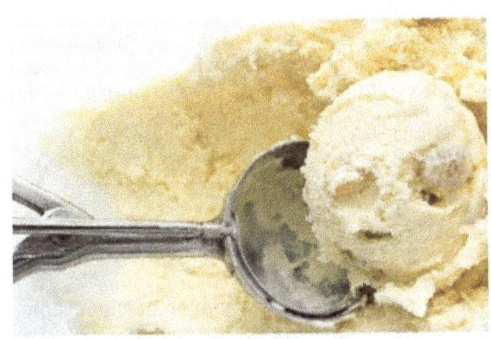

A delicious Guadeloupean specialty, "Banana Flambé Ice Cream" features ripe bananas flambéed with rum and combined with a creamy ice cream base, creating a delightful tropical dessert.

INGREDIENTS

- 2 cups heavy cream
- 1 cup whole milk
- 3/4 cup granulated sugar
- 4 large egg yolks
- 4 ripe bananas, mashed
- 1/4 cup dark rum
- 1 tablespoon butter
- 1/2 teaspoon vanilla extract

DIRECTIONS

1. In a saucepan, heat the sugar, milk, and heavy cream. Heavy cream, milk, and sugar on medium flame.
2. Cook until it simmers. Stir continuously.
3. In another bowl, beat the egg yolks until the mixture turns into custard-like thick consistency.
4. Slowly pour the hot cream mixture into the egg yolks, whisking constantly.
5. Cook the mixture on low flame until it thickens. Cool this mixture at room temperature.
6. In another pan, melt the butter on medium flame. Add the mashed bananas and cook until they become soft and slightly caramelized.
7. Remove the pan from heat and carefully add the rum. Ignite the rum using a long match or lighter, allowing it to flame and burn off the alcohol.
8. Once the flames subside, add the banana mixture to the cooled ice cream base and stir well.
9. Stir in the vanilla extract.
10. Transfer the mixture to an ice cream make churn by following the manufacturer's instructions.
11. Once churned, transfer the Banana Flambé Ice Cream to a container and freeze for several hours until firm.
12. Serve the ice cream in cones or bowls and indulge in the tropical flavors of Guadeloupe.

ICE CREAM

Tropical Fruit Medley Ice Cream— British Virgin Islands

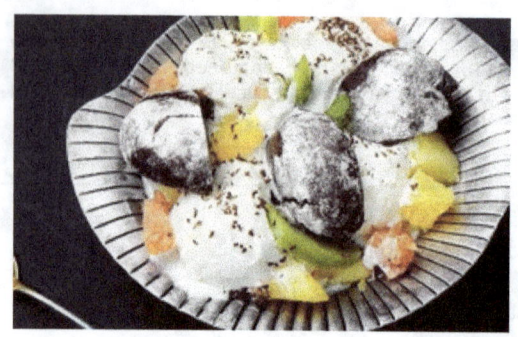

"Tropical Fruit Medley Ice Cream" from the British Virgin Islands celebrates the region's bounty with a blend of exotic fruits and coconut, offering a taste of the Caribbean in every bite.

INGREDIENTS

- 2 cups heavy cream
- 1 cup whole milk
- 3/4 cup granulated sugar
- 4 large egg yolks
- 1 cup mixed tropical fruits (such as mangoes, pineapples, and papayas), diced
- 1/4 cup shredded coconut
- 1 teaspoon lime zest

DIRECTIONS

1. Cook the milk, sugar, and heavy cream on medium flame.
2. In another bowl, beat the egg yolks until custard-like thick Consistency
3. Slowly pour the hot cream mixture into the egg yolks, while stirring continuously.
4. Cook this mixture on low flame, stirring continuously until the mixture thickens.
5. Cool this mixture at room temperature.
6. In a separate bowl, combine the shredded coconut, tropical fruits, and lime zest.
7. Add the fruit mixture to the cooled ice cream base and stir well.
8. Transfer the mixture to an ice cream maker and churn according to the manufacturer's instructions.
9. Once churned, transfer the Tropical Fruit Medley Ice Cream to an airtight container. Freeze for several hours until firm.

SOUTH AMERICA & LATIN AMERICA

ICE CREAM

Exotic Fruit Sorbet — French Guiana

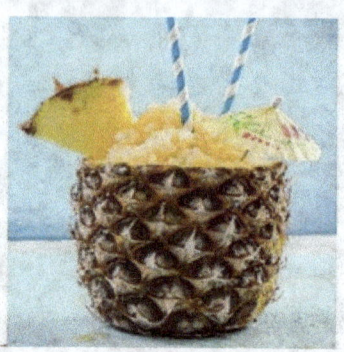

Serve scoops of the ice cream in bowls or cones, and enjoy the tropical flavors of the British Virgin Islands. "Exotic Fruit Sorbet" celebrates the culture of French Guiana, incorporating a blend of passion fruit, guava, and pineapple into a refreshing and fruity sorbet.

INGREDIENTS

- 2 cups mixed exotic fruits (such as passion fruit, guava, and pineapple), pureed
- 1 cup water
- 1 cup sugar
- 1 tablespoon lime juice

DIRECTIONS

1. In a saucepan, combine the sugar and water. Cook until sugar dissolves.
2. Turn off the heat and cool down this sugar syrup at room temperature.
3. In a blender, puree the mixed exotic fruits until smooth.
4. Combine the fruit puree, sugar syrup, and lime juice in a bowl, and mix well.
5. Pour the mixture into an ice cream maker and churn according to the manufacturer's instructions.
6. Once churned, transfer the Exotic Fruit Sorbet to a container and freeze for a few hours until firm.
7. Serve the sorbet in bowls or cones, and savor the refreshing flavors of French Guiana.

ICE CREAM

Horchata Ice Cream — Guatemala

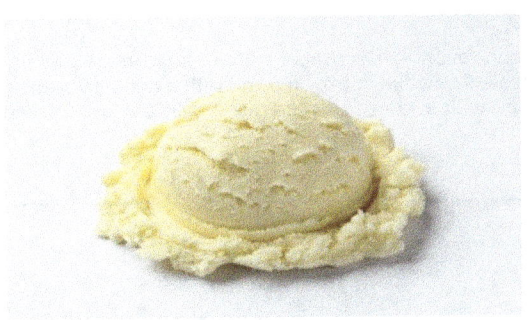

Horchata Ice Cream" from Guatemala features a unique blend of rice milk, cinnamon, and nutmeg, capturing the essence of the traditional horchata beverage in frozen form.

INGREDIENTS

- 2 cups rice milk
- 1 cup heavy cream
- 3/4 cup granulated sugar
- 1/2 teaspoon ground cinnamon
- 1/4 teaspoon ground nutmeg
- 1/2 teaspoon vanilla extract

DIRECTIONS

1. In a saucepan, combine the rice milk, heavy cream, sugar, cinnamon, and nutmeg. Heat over medium heat until it reaches a simmer, stirring occasionally.
2. Remove from heat and stir in the vanilla extract.
3. Allow the mixture to cool completely.
4. Transfer the mixture to an ice cream maker and churn according to the manufacturer's instructions.
5. Once churned, transfer the Horchata Ice Cream to a container and freeze for several hours until firm.
6. Serve scoops of the ice cream in bowls or cones, and enjoy the delightful flavors of Guatemala.

ICE CREAM

TresLeches Ice Cream — Nicaragua

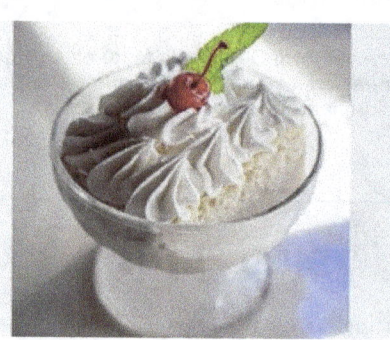

A Nicaraguan favorite, "TresLeches Ice Cream," recreates the beloved tresleches cake in frozen form, with a rich and creamy base infused with sweetened condensed milk and evaporated milk.

INGREDIENTS

- 2 cups heavy cream
- 1 cup whole milk
- 1 can (14 ounces) of sweetened condensed milk
- 1 can (12 ounces) of evaporated milk
- 1 teaspoon vanilla extract

DIRECTIONS

1. In a saucepan, combine the heavy cream, whole milk, sweetened condensed milk, and evaporated milk. Heat over medium heat until it reaches a simmer, stirring occasionally.
2. Remove from heat and stir in the vanilla extract.
3. Allow the mixture to cool completely.
4. Transfer the mixture to an ice cream maker and churn according to the manufacturer's instructions.
5. Once churned, transfer the TresLeches Ice Cream to a container and freeze for several hours until firm.
6. Serve scoops of the ice cream in bowls or cones, and indulge in the creamy goodness of Nicaragua.

NORTH AMERICA

ICE CREAM

Peach Cobbler Ice Cream — Atlanta

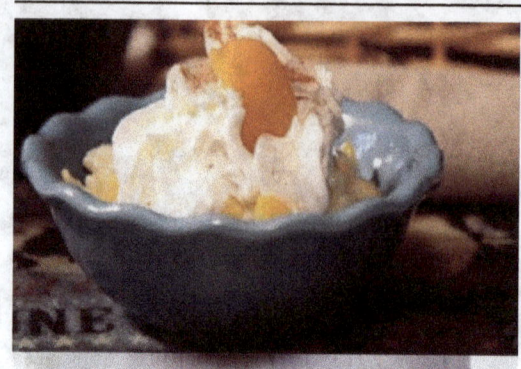

Peach Cobbler Ice Cream" pays homage to the Peach State with a delicious blend of fresh peaches and graham crackers, offering a delightful twist on the classic Southern dessert

INGREDIENTS

- 2 cups heavy cream
- 1 cup whole milk
- 3/4 cup granulated sugar
- 4 large egg yolks
- 2 cups fresh peaches, peeled and diced
- 1 cup crushed graham crackers
- 1 teaspoon vanilla extract
- 1/2 teaspoon ground cinnamon

DIRECTIONS

1. In a saucepan, combine the heavy cream, whole milk, and sugar. Heat over medium heat until it reaches a simmer, stirring occasionally.
2. In a separate bowl, whisk the egg yolks until they become slightly thickened.
3. Slowly pour the hot cream mixture into the egg yolks, whisking constantly.
4. Pour the mixture back into the saucepan and cook over low heat, stirring continuously, until it thickens and coats the back of a spoon.
5. Remove from heat and allow the mixture to cool.
6. In a blender or food processor, puree half of the diced peaches until smooth.
7. Stir the pureed peaches, remaining diced peaches, crushed graham crackers, vanilla extract, and ground cinnamon into the cooled ice cream base.
8. Transfer the mixture to an ice cream maker and churn according to the manufacturer's instructions.
9. Once churned, transfer the Peach Cobbler Ice Cream to a container and freeze for several hours until firm.
10. Serve scoops of the ice cream in bowls or cones, and savor the sweet taste of Atlanta's famous peaches.

ICE CREAM

Maple Pecan Ice Cream— Edmonton

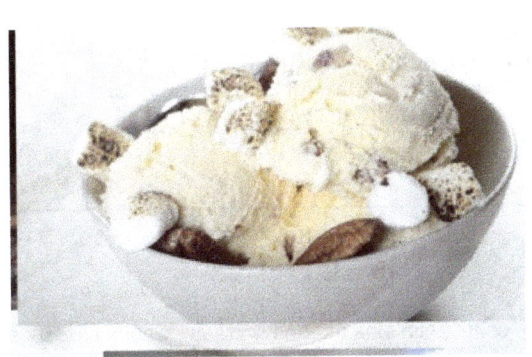

Maple Pecan Ice Cream" from Edmonton showcases the iconic Canadian flavors of maple syrup and toasted pecans, delivering a rich and nutty ice cream experience.

INGREDIENTS

- 2 cups heavy cream
- 1 cup whole milk
- 3/4 cup maple syrup
- 4 large egg yolks
- 1/2 cup chopped pecans
- 1/2 teaspoon vanilla extract

DIRECTIONS

1. In a saucepan, heat the maple syrup, milk, and heavy cream. heavy cream, milk, and sugar on medium flame.
2. Cook until it simmers. Stir continuously.
3. In another bowl, beat the egg yolks until the mixture turns into a custard-like thick consistency.
4. Slowly pour the hot cream mixture into the egg yolks, whisking constantly.
5. Cook the mixture on low flame until it thickens. Add lime juice and zest.
6. Cool this mixture at room temperature.
7. Then churn by following the manufacturer's
8. instructions
9. In a separate pan, toast the chopped pecans over medium heat until they become fragrant and lightly browned. Set aside to cool.
10. Stir the toasted pecans and vanilla extract into the cooled ice cream base.
11. Transfer the mixture to an ice cream maker and churn according to the manufacturer's instructions.
12. Once churned, transfer the Maple Pecan Ice Cream to a container and freeze for several hours until firm.
13. Serve scoops of the ice cream in bowls or cones, and enjoy the delightful combination of maple and pecans.

ICE CREAM

Mango Chamoy Ice Cream – La Paz, Baja California

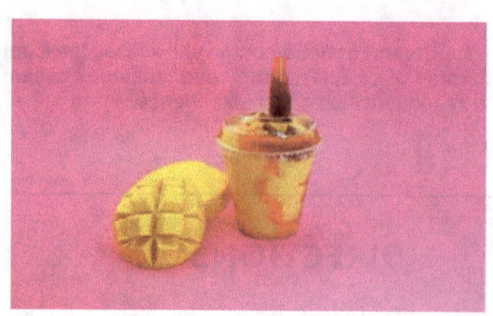

Mango Chamoy Ice Cream" brings a taste of Mexico to the table, blending mango puree with tangy chamoy sauce and a hint of lime for a sweet and spicy treat.

INGREDIENTS

- 2 cups mango puree (fresh or frozen)
- 1 cup heavy cream
- 1 cup whole milk
- 3/4 cup granulated sugar
- 4 large egg yolks
- 1/4 cup
- lime juice 2 teaspoons.
- 2 tablespoons chamoy sauce (a Mexican condiment made from pickled fruit)
- 1 teaspoon Tajin seasoning (a Mexican seasoning blend of chili, lime, and salt)

DIRECTIONS

1. In a saucepan, combine the heavy cream, whole milk, sugar, and mango puree. Heat over medium heat until it reaches a simmer, stirring occasionally.
2. In a separate bowl, whisk the egg yolks until they become slightly thickened.
3. Slowly pour the hot cream mixture into the egg yolks, whisking constantly.
4. Pour the mixture back into the saucepan and cook over low heat, stirring continuously, until it thickens and coats the back of a spoon.
5. Remove from heat and allow the mixture to cool.
6. Stir in the lime juice, chamoy sauce, and Tajin seasoning into the cooled ice cream base. Adjust the amount of chamoy and Tajin seasoning to suit your taste.
7. Transfer the mixture to an ice cream maker and churn according to the manufacturer's instructions.
8. Once churned, transfer the Mango Chamoy Ice Cream to a container and freeze for several hours until firm.
9. Serve scoops of the ice cream in bowls or cones, and enjoy the sweet and tangy flavors of La Paz.

SECTION VII

PUDDINGS

AFRICA

Africa offers a delightful array of puddings that are rich in flavor and steeped in cultural traditions. From Morocco to Egypt and Botswana, each country has its own unique twist on the art of pudding-making, making it an essential part of their holiday feasting.

PUDDINGS

Moroccan Orange Blossom Pudding- Morocco

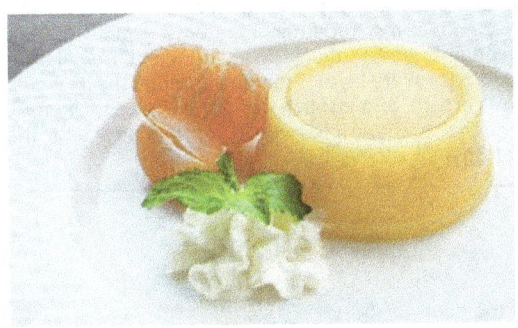

The Kingdom of Morocco is located in North Africa. The Moroccan Orange Blossom Pudding captures the essence of Moroccan cuisine and its love for aromatic ingredients. With each spoonful, you'll experience the joy of this dessert.

INGREDIENTS

- 4 cups Milk
- 1 cup Sugar ▫ 1 pinch Salt
- 1/2 cup Cornstarch
- 1/2 cup Water
- 2 tablespoons Orange Blossom Water
- Orange zest (for garnish)

DIRECTIONS

1. In a saucepan, combine milk, sugar, and a pinch of salt. Cook until it simmers. Keep flame medium.
2. Stir occasionally to dissolve the sugar and prevent sticking. In a separate bowl, whisk together 1/2 cup of cornstarch and 1/2 cup of water until smooth, creating a cornstarch mixture.
3. Slowly pour the cornstarch mixture into the simmering milk while stirring continuously. This step helps thicken the pudding.
4. Keep stirring the mixture constantly until it thickens to a creamy consistency. This may take a few minutes.
5. Remove the saucepan from the heat and stir in 2 tablespoons of orange blossom water. This will infuse the pudding with a delightful orange blossom flavor.
6. Now, it's time to transfer the pudding into individual serving dishes. You can use small bowls, ramekins, or any serving dish of your choice.
7. Allow the pudding to cool down to room temperature before refrigerating it. Once cooled, cover the dishes and place them in the refrigerator.
8. Let the pudding chill in the refrigerator until it sets completely. This may take a few hours, so it's best to leave it in the fridge for at least 2-3 hours or overnight for the best results.
9. When ready to serve, garnish each serving with a sprinkle of orange zest. The orange zest adds a burst of citrus aroma and enhances the overall presentation.
10. Enjoy your Moroccan Orange Blossom Pudding chilled and savor the delicate blend of flavors!
11. Note: You can also customize the recipe by adding sliced fresh oranges or a drizzle of honey on top of the pudding before serving, for extra sweetness and a vibrant touch. Enjoy this delightful dessert as a refreshing and exotic treat!

PUDDINGS

Umm Ali (Egyptian Bread Pudding) — Egypt

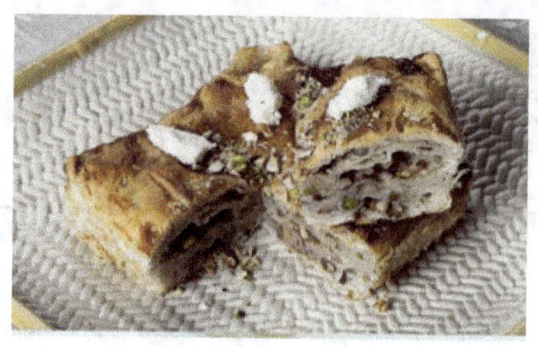

Egypt is the land of pyramids and pharaohs, where history and culinary brilliance come together to create Umm Ali, the beloved Egyptian Bread Pudding. This indulgent treat has a story woven into its every layer. From the crunchy toasted nuts to the luscious cream, and a touch of fragrant spices, Umm Ali is a dessert that carries the weight of legends and the sweetness of Egypt's ancient past.

INGREDIENTS

- 4 cups milk
- 1/2 cup granulated sugar
- 1/2 teaspoon vanilla extract
- 1/2 cup chopped nuts (almonds or pistachios)
- 1/4 cup raisins
- Puff pastry or croissants
- Powdered sugar (for dusting)

DIRECTIONS

1. Preheat the oven to 350°F (175°C).
2. In a saucepan, combine the milk, sugar, and vanilla extract over medium heat.
3. Bring the mixture to a boil, stirring occasionally, and then remove it from the heat.
4. Stir in the chopped nuts and raisins, creating a delightful blend of flavors.
5. In a baking dish, evenly layer pieces of puff pastry or croissants.
6. Pour the milk mixture over the pastry, ensuring it soaks through each layer.
7. Allow the dessert to sit for a few minutes, letting the flavors meld together.
8. Bake in the preheated oven for 20-25 minutes until the top turns golden brown.
9. Once baked to perfection, remove it from the oven and let it cool slightly.
10. Dust the warm Umm Ali with powdered sugar, adding a touch of sweetness.
11. Sprinkle additional chopped nuts on top for an enticing crunch.
12. Serve the Umm Ali warm, savoring the rich and satisfying flavors.
13. Enjoy this traditional Egyptian dessert with your loved ones, and immerse yourself in the history and joy it brings to your table!

PUDDINGS

Malva Pudding — Botswana

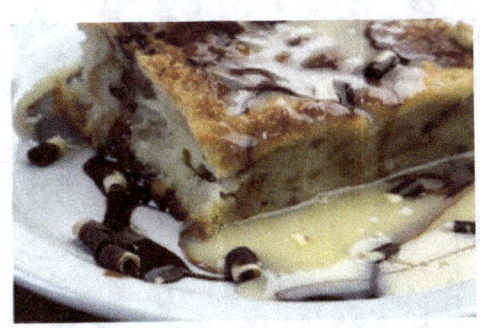

Botswana is a land of untouched wilderness and warm-hearted hospitality. Among the diverse culinary delights, Botswana's beloved Malva Pudding stands out—a delectable sponge cake infused with apricot jam and warm spices, soaked in a velvety caramel sauce. Served warm and symbolizing togetherness, this dessert captures the essence of Botswana's culture, leaving you with sweet memories of this country.

INGREDIENTS

- 1 cup all-purpose flour
- 1 teaspoon baking soda
- Pinch of salt
- 1 large egg
- 1 cup sugar
- 1 tablespoon apricot jam (or apricot jam syrup)
- 1 tablespoon melted butter
- 1 teaspoon vanilla extract
- 1 tablespoon white vinegar
- 1 cup milk

For the Sauce:
- 1 cup heavy cream
- 1 cup sugar
- 1/2 cup butter
- 1/2 cup hot water

DIRECTIONS

1. Preheat your oven to 350°F (175°C). Grease a medium-sized baking dish. sift the all-purpose -flour, baking soda, and salt in a mixing bowl, cover, and set aside for later use.
2. In another bowl, beat the sugar and eggs until creamy and light in texture.
3. Add melted butter, apricot jam, vinegar, vanilla extract, egg, and sugar mixture. Mix all wet ingredients with a spatula.
4. Gradually add the dry ingredients to the wet mixture, alternating with the milk, and mix until you have a smooth batter.
5. Pour batter into a greased and lined baking dish.
6. Bake the pudding in the preheated oven for about 3035 minutes or until a toothpick inserted into the center comes out clean.
7. While the pudding is baking, prepare the sauce. In a saucepan, combine the sugar, butter, heavy cream heavy, and hot water.
8. Boil this mixture, and stir continuously until the sugar dissolves completely.
9. As soon as the pudding is removed from the oven, poke several holes into it using a skewer or fork.
10. Pour the hot sauce over the hot pudding, allowing it to soak in slowly.
11. Leave the pudding for 15 minutes before serving to absorb the sauce well.
12. Serve the Botswana Malva Pudding warm, preferably with a dollop of whipped cream or a scoop of vanilla ice cream for an extra indulgent treat!
13. Enjoy the luscious sweetness and comforting flavors of Botswana Malva Pudding, a true delight that embodies the heartwarming essence of Botswana's dessert cuisine.

ASIA

PUDDINGS

Kheer — Pakistan

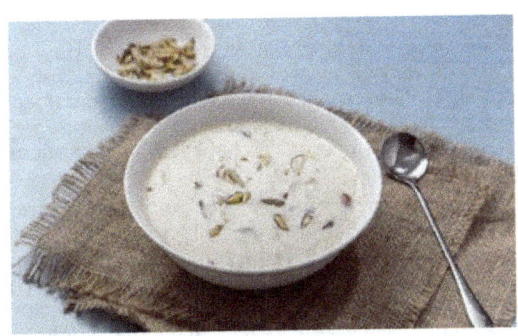

Located in South Asia, Pakistan has a rich culinary heritage with a blend of flavors and traditional desserts. Kheer is a creamy rice pudding infused with cardamom and garnished with nuts and saffron. It is often served during Eid celebrations, weddings, and other festive occasions.

INGREDIENTS

- 1/2 cup basmati rice
- 4 cups whole milk
- 1/2 cup sugar
- 1/4 cup mixed dry fruits (almonds, raisins, pistachios, almonds or cashews), chopped
- 1/4 teaspoon cardamom powder
- A pinch of saffron strands (optional)

DIRECTIONS

1. Wash the basmati rice in cold water and drain it.
2. In a large saucepan, bring the whole milk to a boil over medium heat.
3. Add the rinsed rice to the boiling milk and let it simmer on low heat. Stir occasionally to prevent sticking.
4. After approximately 30 minutes, the rice will be cooked and the mixture will thicken.
5. Stir in the sugar, cardamom powder, and saffron strands (if using), ensuring the sugar dissolves.
6. Continue cooking for another 5-10 minutes until the kheer reaches the desired consistency.
7. Remove the saucepan from the heat and let the kheer cool down.
8. Before serving, garnish the kheer with the chopped nuts. It can be served warm or chilled, making it a delightful addition to holiday festivities.

PUDDINGS

Bubur Cha Cha — Malaysia

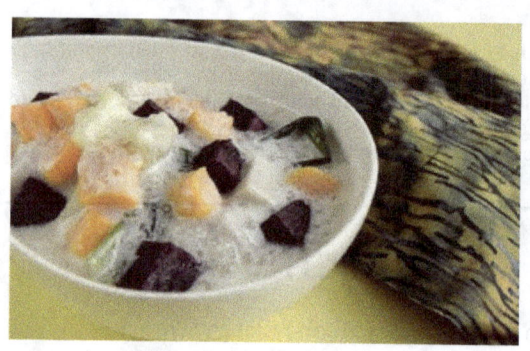

A melting pot of cultures, Malaysia offers an array of delectable desserts for holiday festivities. "Bubur Cha Cha" is a favorite during festive seasons, featuring sweet potatoes, taro, and sago pearls cooked in coconut milk and palm sugar. This colorful and flavorful dessert is cherished by Malaysians of all backgrounds.

INGREDIENTS

- 1 sweet potato, peeled and diced
- 1 taro root, peeled and diced
- 1/4 cup sago pearls
- 1 can (400ml) coconut milk
- 1/2 cup palm sugar (gula Melaka), grated
- A pinch of salt

DIRECTIONS

1. Start by boiling the diced sweet potato and taro separately in two different pots until they become tender. Then, drain and set them aside.
2. In another saucepan, cook the sago pearls in boiling water until they turn translucent. Drain the sago pearls and set them aside as well.
3. In a larger saucepan, combine the coconut milk, grated palm sugar, and a pinch of salt. Stir the mixture over low heat until the palm sugar dissolves and the mixture slightly thickens.
4. Add the cooked sweet potato, taro, and sago pearls into the coconut milk mixture. Mix well.
5. Allow the mixture to simmer for a few more minutes, allowing the flavors to blend.
6. You can now serve the Bubur Cha Cha warm or chilled in individual bowls, making it a delightful treat for holiday celebrations

PUDDINGS

Serradura — Macau

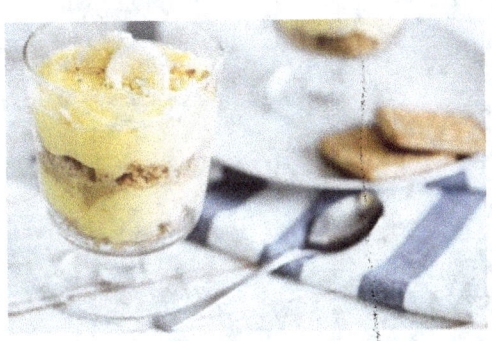

As a fusion of Chinese and Portuguese cultures, Macau's holiday feastings are graced with unique sweet treats. "Serradura" or sawdust pudding is a popular dessert made with layers of sweetened condensed milk and crushed biscuits, creating a delightful and creamy delicacy enjoyed during festive gatherings

INGREDIENTS

- 200g tea biscuits (such as Marie biscuits or similar)
- 1 can (395g) sweetened condensed milk
- 250ml whipping cream
- 1 teaspoon vanilla extract

DIRECTIONS

1. Start by crushing the tea biscuits into fine crumbs. You can do this by using a food processor or placing the biscuits in a plastic bag and rolling a rolling pin over them.
2. In a mixing bowl, whip the whipping cream and vanilla extract until soft peaks form. This means the cream will be thickened, but still airy.
3. Gently fold the sweetened condensed milk into the whipped cream until everything is well combined. This will create a creamy and sweet mixture.
4. Now, it's time to assemble the dessert. You can use serving glasses or a large dish for this. Begin by layering the biscuit crumbs and the cream mixture alternately. Start with a layer of biscuit crumbs, then add a layer of the cream mixture. Repeat this process, finishing with a layer of biscuit crumbs on top.
5. Once everything is layered, refrigerate the dessert for at least 2-3 hours before serving. This chilling time allows the flavors to come together and creates a delicious, cohesive dessert.
6. Just before serving, you can garnish the Serradura with a sprinkle of biscuit crumbs on top for a nice finishing touch. Enjoy this delightful Macanese dessert during festive occasions or any time you're craving a sweet treat!

AUSTRALIA & OCEANIA

PUDDINGS

Pavlova — Papua New Guinea

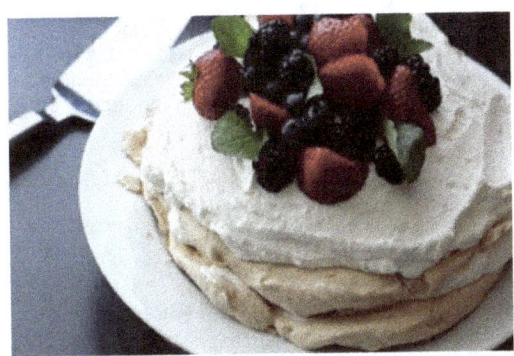

Across the diverse nations of Australia and Oceania, holiday feasts feature an assortment of puddings and sweet delicacies. One iconic dessert is the "Pavlova," a meringue-based cake topped with fresh fruits such as kiwi, passion fruit, and berries. It is a centerpiece during celebratory occasions

INGREDIENTS

- 4 large egg whites, at room temperature
- 1 cup caster sugar
- 1 teaspoon white vinegar
- 1 teaspoon cornstarch
- 1 teaspoon vanilla extract
- Fresh fruits (kiwi, berries, passion fruit) for topping
- Whipped cream for serving

DIRECTIONS

1. Preheat your oven to 120°C (250°F) and prepare a baking tray blining it with parchment paper.
2. In a clean mixing bowl, use an electric mixer to beat the egg whites until soft peaks form. This means the egg whites will be fluffy and hold their shape when the beaters are lifted.
3. Gradually add the caster sugar to the egg whites, one spoonful at a time, while continuing to beat. Keep beating until the mixture becomes glossy and stiff peaks form. Stiff peaks mean that the mixture will stand upright and won't flop over when the beaters are lifted.
4. Gently fold in the white vinegar, cornstarch, and vanilla extract until everything is fully mixed. This helps stabilize the meringue and gives it a chewy interior. Spoon the meringue mixture onto the prepared baking tray, shaping it into a round nest with a slight indentation in the middle. The indentation will hold the toppings later.
5. Bake the pavlova for about 1.5 to 2 hours, or until the outside is crisp and dry, while the inside remains marshmallow-like. A longer baking time will create a crisper exterior.
6. Once baked, let the pavlova cool completely in the oven with the door slightly ajar. This gradual cooling prevents cracking.
7. Just before serving, top the pavlova with fresh fruits like kiwi, berries, or passion fruit. Top with whipped cream.
8. Slice and enjoy this delightful and light dessert during festive gatherings or any special occasion. The combination of crunchy meringue, creamy whipped cream, and fresh fruits is simply irresistible!

PUDDINGS

Saksak — Papua New Guinea

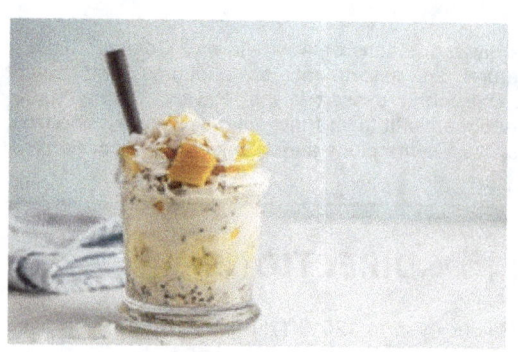

In the tropical paradise of Papua New Guinea, celebrations are accompanied by unique desserts like "Saksak." Made from mashed bananas and sweet potatoes, this delicious pudding is wrapped in banana leaves and cooked in an earth oven, delighting taste buds with its natural sweetness.

INGREDIENTS

- 2 ripe bananas
- 1 cup grated sweet potato
- 1 cup grated cassava
- 1 cup grated taro ⊠ 1 cup grated yam
- 1 cup grated pumpkin
- Banana leaves for wrapping

DIRECTIONS

1. Begin by mashing the ripe bananas in a large mixing bowl.
2. Add the grated sweet potato, cassava, taro, yam, and pumpkin to the mashed bananas. Mix everything thoroughly until well combined.
3. Cut the banana leaves into rectangular pieces and gently pass them over an open flame to soften them.
4. Take a scoop of the mixed grated vegetables and place it in the center of a piece of banana leaf.
5. Fold the banana leaf over the vegetable mixture to create a small packet, and secure the edges using toothpicks or string.
6. Steam the packets in a steamer for about 30-40 minutes until the mixture is thoroughly cooked and set.
7. To serve the Saksak, present it warm during holiday celebrations, and unwrap the banana leaves to reveal the delightful flavors

PUDDINGS

Pavlova - A Classic New Zealand Dessert

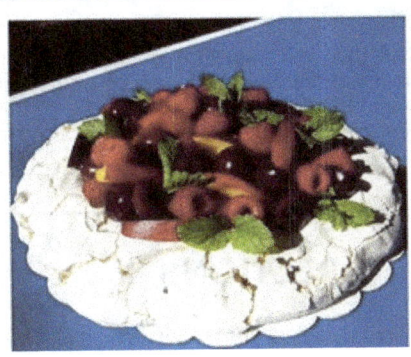

Pavlova is a popular and iconic New Zealand dessert, named after the Russian ballerina Anna Pavlova. It's a meringue-based dessert with a crisp outer shell and a soft, marshmallow-like interior, usually topped with whipped cream and fresh fruits.

INGREDIENTS

- 4 large egg whites, at room temperature
- 1 cup caster sugar (superfine sugar)
- 1 teaspoon cornstarch (corn flour)
- 1 teaspoon white vinegar
- 1/2 teaspoon vanilla extract
- 1 cup heavy cream
- 2 tablespoons powdered sugar
- Fresh fruits (kiwifruit, strawberries, passion fruit, or any other berries) for topping

DIRECTIONS

1. Preheat your oven to 300°F (150°C)
2. Line a baking sheet with butter paper.
3. In a clean, dry mixing bowl, whisk the egg whites with an electric mixer on medium-high speed until soft peaks form.
4. Add 1/4 cup sugar at a time. Keep mixing at high speed.
5. Make sure the sugar is fully dissolved, and the mixture is thick and glossy.
6. Reduce the mixer speed to low and gently fold in the cornstarch, white vinegar, and vanilla extract.
7. Spoon the meringue onto the prepared baking sheet, shaping it into a circle or any desired shape, with slightly raised edges.
8. Put the baking sheet into the oven that has been preheated, then promptly lower the temperature to 250°F (120°C
9. Bake for about 1 hour to 1 hour 15 minutes, or until the pavlova is crisp on the outside and slightly ivory colored.
10. Turn off the oven and leave the Pavlova inside to cool completely with the oven door slightly ajar.
11. In a separate mixing bowl, whip the heavy cream and powdered sugar until it reaches a thick and fluffy consistency.
12. Carefully transfer the cooled Pavlova to a serving plate. Top it with whipped cream and decorate with fresh fruits.
13. Serve the delicious Pavlova immediately or refrigerate for a short while to chill before serving. Enjoy this delightful New Zealand dessert!
14. Ensure that all equipment used to whip the egg whites and cream is clean and free of any grease, as it can hinder proper whipping

PUDDINGS

Boysenberry Fool — Cook Islands

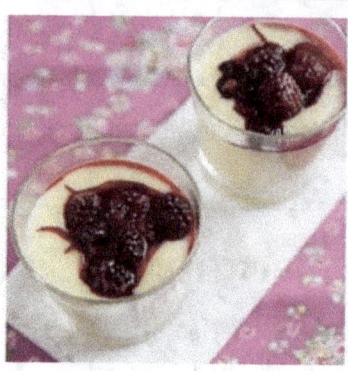

Cook Islands offer the delicious "Boysenberry Fool" as a holiday treat. This delightful dessert combines boysenberries with whipped cream, creating a light and refreshing pudding perfect for warm-weather festivities.

INGREDIENTS

- 2 cups fresh boysenberries (or any other berries)
- 1/4 cup granulated sugar (adjust to taste)
- 1 cup heavy cream
- 1 tablespoon powdered sugar
- 1 teaspoon vanilla extract

DIRECTIONS

1. In a saucepan, combine the fresh boysenberries and granulated sugar over low heat. Cook the berries until they soften and release their juices, creating a berry compote. Allow it to cool completely.
2. In a separate mixing bowl, whip the heavy cream, powdered sugar, and vanilla extract until soft peaks form.
3. Gently fold the cooled berry compote into the whipped cream, creating a marbled effect.
4. Spoon the Boysenberry Fool into individual dessert glasses or a large serving dish.
5. Refrigerate the dessert for at least 1-2 hours before serving during festive occasions. Enjoy!

EUROPE

PUDDINGS

Christmas Pudding — United Kingdom

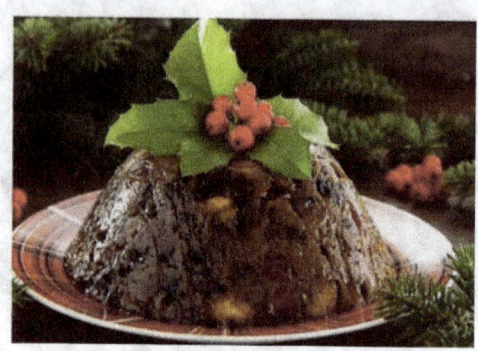

"Christmas Pudding" is an iconic dessert in the UK, filled with dried fruits, spices, and suet. It is often served with a generous splash of brandy or rum and set ablaze before indulging in its rich flavors

INGREDIENTS

- 1 cup mixed dried fruits (raisins, currants, and sultanas)
- 1/2 cup candied peel
- 1/2 cup chopped dried apricots
  1/2 cup chopped prunes
- 1/2 cup brandy or rum 3/4 cup self-raising flour 1/2 cup fresh breadcrumbs 1/2 cup vegetarian suet (or regular suet) 1/2 cup brown sugar 1 teaspoon mixed spice (cinnamon, nutmeg, allspice) Zest of 1 lemon and 1 orange 2 large eggs, beaten 1/4 cup milk

DIRECTIONS

1. In a large mixing bowl, combine the mixed dried fruits, candied peel, apricots, and prunes. Pour the brandy or rum over the fruits and allow them to soak overnight.
2. The next day, add the self-raising flour, breadcrumbs, suet, brown sugar, mixed spice, and citrus zest to the soaked fruits. Mix everything together thoroughly.
3. Stir in the beaten eggs and milk to create a thick, moist batter.
4. Pour this mixture into the greased pudding basin. Cover the basin with parchment paper and aluminum foil, securing them with string.
5. Steam the pudding in a large pot with a lid for approximately 6 hours, making sure to keep the water level topped up.
6. Allow the pudding to cool completely, then rewrap it and store it in a cool, dark place until Christmas Day.
7. To serve, reheat the pudding by steaming it for an additional 2 hours. Remove the wrappings, turn them onto a plate, and garnish with a sprig of holly on top.
8. As a traditional touch, flambé the Christmas pudding with brandy or rum before serving.

PUDDINGS

Tarta de Santiago — Spain

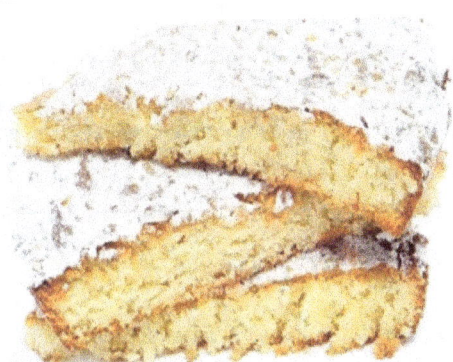

Tarta de Santiago" is a beloved almond cake originating from the Spanish region of Galicia. Embellished with the cross of Saint James, this dessert is cherished during special occasions like Christmas and pilgrimages to Santiago de Compostela.

INGREDIENTS

- 1 1/2 cups ground almonds
- 1 cup granulated sugar
- Zest of 1 lemon
- 4 large eggs
- 1/4 cup unsalted butter,
- Melted Powdered sugar, for dusting

DIRECTIONS

1. Preheat the oven to 180°C for a minimum 15 minutes.
2. Grease and line the cake pan with butter paper or parchment paper.
3. In a mixing bowl, combine the ground almonds, granulated sugar, and lemon zest.
4. Add egg and beat until all well combined. Mix well after adding each egg.
5. Stir in the melted butter until the batter is smooth and well combined.
6. Pour the batter into the prepared cake pan smooth the top with a spatula.
7. Bake for approximately 30-35 minutes or until the top is golden and a toothpick inserted into the center comes out clean.
8. Allow the Tarta de Santiago to cool in the pan for a few minutes before transferring it to a wire rack to cool completely.
9. Once cooled, dust the top of the cake with powdered sugar in the shape of the Cross of Saint James (a sword-shaped cross).
10. Serve this delicious almond cake during special occasions and holiday celebrations

PUDDINGS

Balkava — Greece

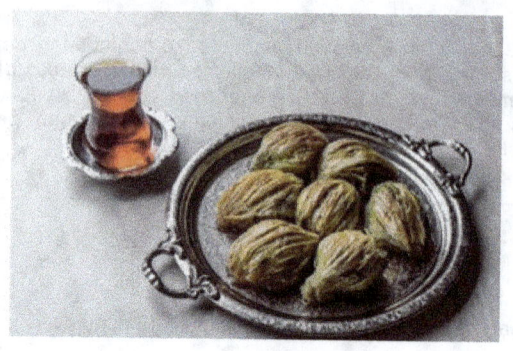

Greek Baklava is a delicious dessert hailing from Greece, made with layers of delicate phyllo pastry sheets, mixed nuts (such as walnuts, pistachios, and almonds) seasoned with ground cinnamon, and a sweet syrup infused with honey and vanilla.

INGREDIENTS

- 1 package (16 oz.) of phyllo pastry sheets
- 2 cups of mixed dry fruits (almonds, walnuts, raisins, pistachios), finely chopped
- 1 teaspoon of ground cinnamon
- 1 cup of unsalted butter, melted
- 1 cup of granulated sugar
- 1 cup of water
- 1/2 cup of honey
- 1 teaspoon of vanilla extract

DIRECTIONS

1. Preheat your oven to 180°C (350°F) and grease a baking dish generously with the melted butter.
2. In a bowl, combine the finely chopped mixed nuts with the ground cinnamon, making a delightful nutty mixture.
3. Carefully unroll the phyllo pastry sheets and trim them to fit the size of your baking dish.
4. Begin layering the phyllo sheets in the dish, brushing each layer with melted butter as you go. Aim for about half of the phyllo sheets to be used in this process.
5. Spread the nut mixture evenly over the buttered phyllo layers, creating a delightful nutty filling.
6. Continue layering the remaining phyllo sheets on top, ensuring to brush each layer with melted butter as before.
7. With a sharp knife, gently cut the baklava into either diamond or square shapes.
8. Bake the baklava in the preheated oven for approximately 45-50 minutes or until it becomes beautifully golden brown and crisp.
9. While the baklava is baking, prepare the sweet syrup. For making sugar syrup, mix the water, sugar , honey, and vanilla
10. Boil this mixture and simmer it on low flame until it thickens. The sugar syrup will be shiny due to the honey and honey will make this dessert irresistible and mind blowing!
11. Once the baklava is out of the oven, immediately pour the hot syrup evenly over it, ensuring that all the pieces are covered with its sweet goodness.
12. Allow the baklava to cool and absorb the syrup thoroughly before serving. This delightful dessert is perfect for special occasions and holiday gatherings, guaranteed to impress your guests with its heavenly flavors. Enjoy!

CARIBBEAN

PUDDINGS

Coconut rice pudding— Anguilla

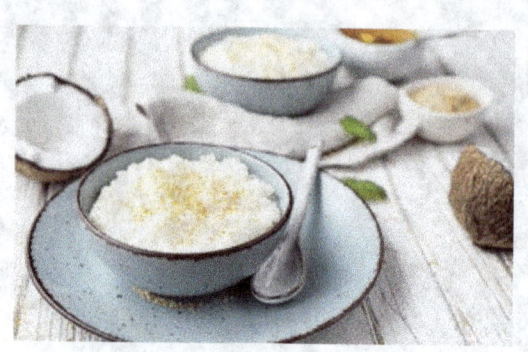

Get a taste of the Caribbean with Anguilla's coconut rice pudding, a popular dessert that adds a tropical twist to holiday feastings. This creamy and rich delicacy combines the warmth of traditional rice pudding with exotic flavors of coconut, aromatic spices, and a hint of vanilla. Served warm or chilled, topped with toasted coconut flakes or fresh tropical fruit, the pudding becomes a visually stunning centerpiece that delights taste buds, making celebrations in Anguilla truly unforgettable.

INGREDIENTS

- 1 cup Arborio rice.
- 2 cups coconut milk
- 1 cup whole milk
- 1/2 cup sugar
- 1/2 cup sweetened shredded coconut
- 1 teaspoon vanilla extract
- 1/2 teaspoon ground cinnamon
- 1/4 teaspoon ground nutmeg
- Pinch of salt
- Optional toppings: toasted coconut flakes, cinnamon, or fresh tropical fruit

DIRECTIONS

1. In a medium-sized saucepan, combine the Arborio rice, coconut milk, whole milk, sugar, shredded coconut, vanilla extract, ground cinnamon, ground nutmeg, and a pinch of salt.
2. Place the saucepan over medium heat and bring the mixture to a gentle simmer, stirring frequently to prevent sticking or burning.
3. Once the mixture is simmering, reduce the heat to low and let it cook uncovered for about 30-35 minutes or until the rice is tender and the pudding has thickened to your desired consistency. Stir continuously.
4. Taste the pudding and adjust the sweetness or spices according to your preference.
5. Once the pudding has reached the desired consistency, remove the saucepan from the heat and allow it to cool slightly.
6. Serve the coconut rice pudding warm in individual dessert bowls. You can sprinkle some toasted coconut flakes, and a dash of cinnamon, or garnish with fresh tropical fruit like mango or pineapple to enhance the presentation and flavor.
7. Enjoy this delectable coconut rice pudding with your loved ones during your holiday celebrations!
8. Note: You can also chill the pudding in the refrigerator if you prefer to serve it cold. It's a versatile dessert

PUDDINGS

Tembleque — Puerto Rico

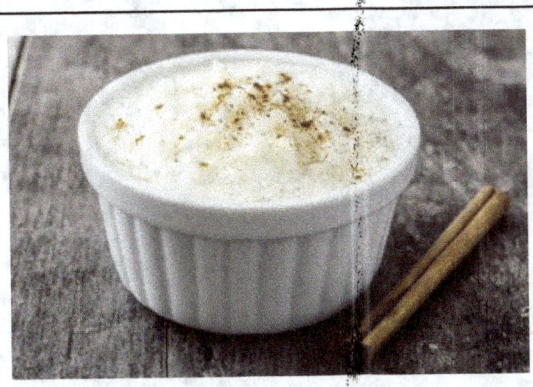

It will add a touch of elegance to your holiday feasting. Tembleque is a traditional Puerto Rican coconut pudding that is both creamy and refreshing, making it the perfect dessert to complement a festive spread. It's named after the Spanish word "temblar," which means "to tremble" or "to shake," referring to its delicate, trembling texture. Let's dive into this holiday treat:

INGREDIENTS

- 1 cup coconut milk
- 2 cups whole milk
- 1/2 cup granulated sugar
- 1/2 cup cornstarch
- 1/4 teaspoon salt
- 1 teaspoon vanilla extract
- Ground cinnamon or shredded coconut (for garnish)

DIRECTIONS

1. In a medium saucepan, combine the coconut milk, whole milk, sugar, cornstarch, and salt. Stir the mixture continuously until the cornstarch dissolves completely.
2. Boil the mixture on medium flame.
3. Then simmer on low flame.
4. Then cook on the stove. Stir continuously to prevent any lumps on the mixture.
5. Cook until the mixture thickens. It must be custardlike consistency.
6. Stir in the vanilla extract, and once fully incorporated, remove the saucepan from the heat.
7. Pour the pudding into large-sized bowls or serving dishes.
8. Allow the pudding to cool for a few minutes at room temperature, then cover it with plastic wrap directly touching the surface to prevent a skin from forming.
9. Refrigerate the Tembleque for at least 2-3 hours or until it sets completely.
10. Before serving, sprinkle some ground cinnamon or shredded coconut on top for a lovely garnish and added flavor.
11. Tembleque velvety smoothness and delightful coconut flavor make it a memorable addition to any holiday celebration.
12. Its simplicity in preparation allows you to focus on other dishes while still wowing your guests with this tropical delight. So, enjoy this Puerto Rican classic and let it bring a taste of the Caribbean to your festive feastings!

SOUTH AMERICA & LATIN AMERICA

PUDDINGS

Bojo – Suriname

Nestled on the northeastern coast of South America, boasts a rich cultural heritage, blending indigenous, African, Indian, and Dutch influences. During holiday feastings, Surinamese households cherish "Bojo," a delectable coconut and cassava pudding. This sweet treat is made with grated cassava, coconut milk, brown sugar, and spices like cinnamon and nutmeg. Baked to perfection, Bojo is a must-have dessert during festive occasions.

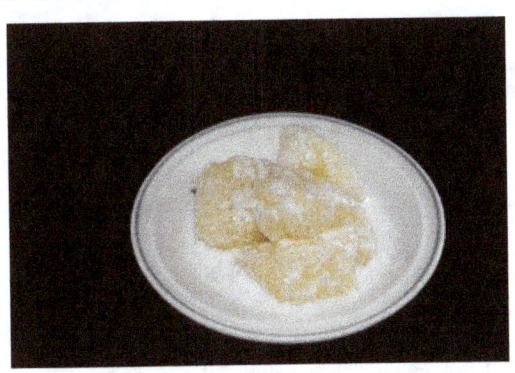

INGREDIENTS

- 1 pound (450g) grated cassava
- 1 can (14 oz.) coconut milk
- 1 cup brown sugar
- 1/2 cup melted butter
- 1 teaspoon ground cinnamon
- 1/2 teaspoon ground nutmeg
- 1/2 teaspoon vanilla extract
- A pinch of salt
- Optional garnish: Raisins and almond flakes

DIRECTIONS

1. Preheat the oven to 350°F (175°C) and grease a baking dish to prepare for baking.
2. In a large mixing bowl, combine the grated cassava, coconut milk, brown sugar, melted butter, ground cinnamon, ground nutmeg, vanilla extract, and a pinch of salt. Mix well.
3. Pour the mixture into the greased baking dish, spreading it out evenly.
4. Optionally, you can garnish the top with raisins and almond flakes for added visual appeal and flavor.
5. Place the Bojo in the preheated oven and bake for approximately 1 hour or until the top turns a golden brown color, and the edges become crispy.
6. Once baked, remove the Bojo from the oven and allow it to cool slightly before serving.
7. Cut the Bojo into squares for easy serving, and delight in this delicious Surinamese pudding during your special holiday feasts.
8. Enjoy the unique flavors and rich texture of this delightful Surinamese dessert!

PUDDINGS

Curacao pudding — Curacao

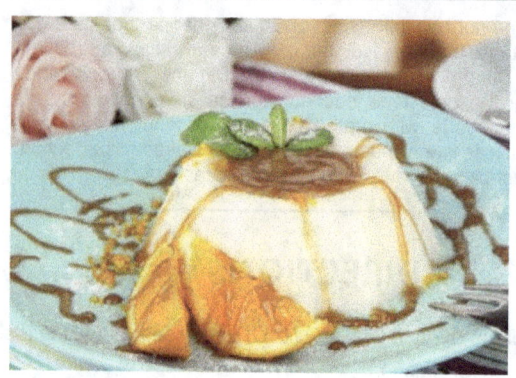

Curacao pudding is a delightful dessert that combines the flavors of the Caribbean with a creamy, refreshing texture.

INGREDIENTS

- 1 cup granulated sugar
- 1/2 cup cornstarch
- 1/4 teaspoon salt
- 4 cups milk
- 4 large egg yolks
- 1 tablespoon unsalted butter
- Orange slices or zest (1 orange.)
- 2 tablespoons Blue Curacao liqueur
- (optional, for flavor and color)
- Whipped cream (optional, for serving)
- Orange slices or zest (for garnish)

DIRECTIONS

1. In a medium-sized saucepan, whisk together the sugar, cornstarch, and salt until well combined.
2. In a separate bowl, whisk the egg yolks until they are smooth and well-beaten.
3. Gradually add the milk to the dry ingredients in the saucepan, stirring constantly to avoid lumps.
4. Place the saucepan on medium heat and cook the mixture, stirring constantly, until it thickens and begins to boil. This should take about 8-10 minutes.
5. Take a small amount of the hot mixture and slowly add it to the beaten egg yolks while stirring vigorously. This process helps to temper the yolks, preventing them from curdling when added to the hot mixture.
6. Gradually pour the tempered egg yolks into the saucepan while stirring continuously.
7. Return the saucepan to the stove and cook the mixture on low heat for an additional 2-3 minutes, stirring constantly, until it reaches a pudding-like consistency.
8. Remove the saucepan from the heat and stir in the unsalted butter, orange zest, and Blue Curacao liqueur (if using). The Blue Curacao will give the pudding a beautiful blue color, reminiscent of the Caribbean seas.
9. Allow the pudding to cool to room temperature before transferring it to individual serving dishes or a large bowl.
10. Cover the pudding with plastic wrap, ensuring the wrap touches the surface of the pudding to prevent skin from forming.
11. When ready to serve, garnish with whipped cream and fresh orange slices or zest.
12. Enjoy your delightful Curacao pudding, a taste of the Caribbean in every spoonful! Remember, you can adjust the sweetness and flavor by adding more or less sugar or Blue Curacao according to your preference.

PUDDINGS

Budín de Pan — Paraguay

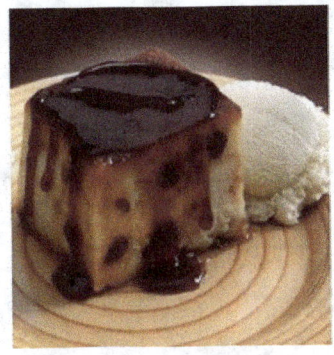

For holiday feasting in Paraguay, "Budín de Pan" is a popular and delightful bread pudding that makes for a perfect dessert.

INGREDIENTS

- 8 cups stale bread, cut into small cubes

(French or any white bread works well)

- 4 cups whole milk
- 1 cup granulated sugar
- 4 large eggs
- 1 tablespoon vanilla extract
- 1/2 cup raisins (optional)
- 1/2 cup chopped dry fruits (such as walnuts or almonds) (optional)
- 1 teaspoon ground cinnamon
- Pinch of sal
- Butter or oil for greasing the baking dish
- For the Caramel Sauce (optional but delicious):
- 1 cup granulated sugar
- 1/4 cup water

DIRECTIONS

1. Preheat your oven to 180°C (350°F). Grease a large baking dish (approximately 9x13 inches) with butter or oil.
2. First of all, heat milk on medium flame until it simmers. Then Cool it at room temperature.
3. In a large mixing bowl, combine the eggs, sugar, vanilla extract, ground cinnamon, and a pinch of salt. Whisk everything together until well combined.
4. Slowly pour the warm milk into the egg mixture while continuously whisking to avoid curdling the eggs.
5. Add the cubed bread to the mixture and let it soak for about 15-20 minutes, allowing the bread to absorb the liquid.
6. If using, fold in the raisins and chopped nuts into the bread mixture.
7. Pour the bread pudding mixture into the greased baking dish and ensure it is evenly distributed.
8. Bake in the preheated oven for approximately 45-55 minutes or until the top is golden brown, and the pudding is set. You can check for doneness by inserting a toothpick into the center; it should come out clean when it's ready.
9. While the bread pudding is baking, you can prepare the caramel sauce (optional). In a separate saucepan, combine the sugar and water over medium-high heat.
10. Let it cook without stirring until the sugar turns into a golden caramel color. Be careful not to burn it. Turn off the heat immediately when it's ready.
11. When the bread pudding is done baking, remove it from the oven and let it cool slightly. If you're using caramel sauce, drizzle it over the warm bread pudding.
12. You can serve the Budín de Pan warm or at room temperature. Some people enjoy it with a scoop of vanilla ice cream or a dollop of whipped cream for an extra special treat.
13. Budín de Pan is a beloved dessert in Paraguay, especially during holiday feasts. Its sweet, custardy texture and comforting flavors make it a delightful ending to a festive meal. Enjoy!

NORTH AMERICA

PUDDINGS

Coconut Tapioca Pudding — Miami, Florida

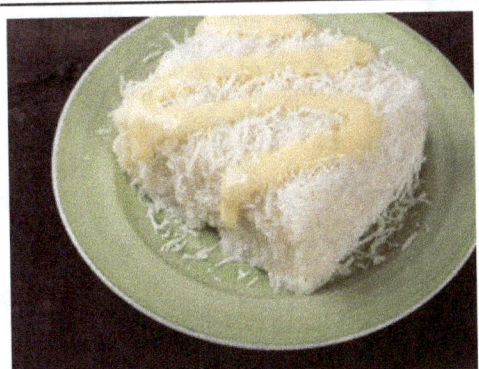

Experience the essence of Miami, Florida, with the delightful Coconut Tapioca Pudding—a creamy tropical fusion of small tapioca pearls simmered in coconut milk and whole milk, sweetened with granulated sugar, and flavored with a touch of vanilla extract.

INGREDIENTS

- 1/2 cup small tapioca pearls
- 2 1/2 cups coconut milk (canned or fresh)
- 1/2 cup whole milk
- 1/2 cup granulated sugar
- 1/4 teaspoon salt
- 1 teaspoon vanilla extract
- 1/2 cup sweetened and toasted shredded coconut for garnishing.
- Fresh fruit (such as mango, pineapple, or berries, for garnish)

DIRECTIONS

1. Wash the tapioca pearls under tap water and drain them.
2. In a medium-sized saucepan, combine the rinsed tapioca pearls, coconut milk, whole milk, granulated sugar, and salt.
3. Simmer this mixture on low flame. Stir continuously to prevent burning or sticking of the mixture to the bottom.
4. Simmer until the tapioca pearls become soft
5. Stir in the vanilla extract and remove the pudding from the heat.
6. Allow the pudding to cool to room temperature before transferring it to individual serving bowls or a large serving dish.
7. Cover the pudding with plastic wrap, ensuring the wrap touches the surface of the pudding to prevent skin from forming.
8. Refrigerate the coconut tapioca pudding for at least 2 hours or until chilled and set.
9. Before serving, toast the sweetened shredded coconut in a dry skillet over medium heat until it turns golden brown and fragrant.
10. To serve, top each portion of pudding with a sprinkle of toasted coconut and fresh fruit for a tropical and delightful Miami-inspired holiday pudding.
11. Enjoy this creamy and coco nutty tapioca pudding as a sweet and refreshing addition to your holiday feastings in Miami, Florida

PUDDINGS

Butter Tart Pudding — Ottawa, Canada

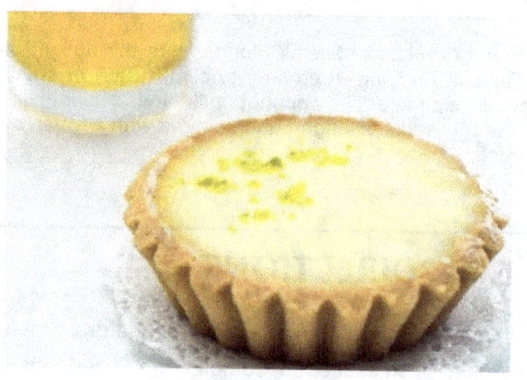

As the capital of Canada, Ottawa embraces a rich culinary diversity. One traditional pudding that graces the holiday feasts is "Butter Tart Pudding." These mini-pastries are made with a buttery and flaky pastry shell, filled with a mixture of butter, brown sugar, and raisins or pecans. Baked until the filling caramelizes, these tarts add a sweet touch to the festive celebrations in Ottawa.

INGREDIENTS

- 1 1/4 cups all-purpose flour
- 1/4 cup granulated sugar
- 1/2 cup unsalted butter, cold and cubed
- 1 large egg yolk ⊠ 1-2 tablespoons cold water
- For the filling:
- 1/2 cup unsalted butter, melted
- 1 cup brown sugar, packed
- 1/4 cup maple syrup
- 2 large eggs
- 1 teaspoon vanilla extract
- 1/4 cup raisins or chopped pecans (optional) Instructions: For the pastry:

DIRECTIONS

1. In a food processor, combine the flour and granulated sugar. Add the cold butter and pulse until the mixture achieves a texture resembling coarse crumbs.
2. Add the egg yolk and pulse again. Gradually add the cold water, one tablespoon at a time, while pulsing, until the dough comes together and forms a ball.
3. Gently shape the dough into a disc, then wrap it in plastic wrap and refrigerate for 1/2 hour.
4. For the filling: 4. Preheat your oven to 375°F (190°C).
5. In a mixing bowl, whisk together the melted butter, brown sugar, maple syrup, eggs, and vanilla extract until well combined.
6. If desired, stir in the raisins or chopped pecans into the filling mixture.
7. Assembling the Butter Tart Pudding: 7. On a lightly floured surface, roll out the chilled pastry dough to fit a 9-inch pie dish. Press the dough into the dish, trimming any excess from the edges.
8. Pour the prepared filling into the pastry shell.
9. Baking the Butter Tart Pudding: 9. Bake the pudding in the preheated oven for about 20-25 minutes or until the filling is set and the pastry is golden brown.
10. Discard from the oven. Cool it at room temperature before slicing.
11. Optionally, serve with a dollop of whipped cream or a scoop of vanilla ice cream for a delightful Canadian holiday treat.

PUDDINGS

Arroz con Leche – CAMPECHE Mexico

Campeche is located on the coast of the Yucatán Peninsula. Arroz con Leche." This classic dish, made with tender white rice, velvety whole milk, and infused with the warmth of cinnamon, offers a taste of nostalgia and comfort.

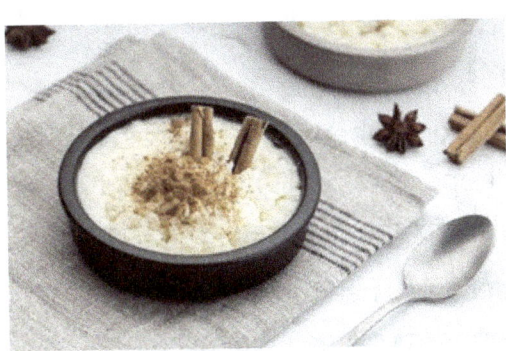

INGREDIENTS

- 1 cup short or medium-grain white rice
- 4 cups whole milk
- 1 cinnamon stick
- 1/2 cup granulated sugar (adjust to taste)
- 1/4 teaspoon salt
- 1 teaspoon vanilla extract
- Ground cinnamon, for garnish

DIRECTIONS

1. Begin by rinsing the white rice thoroughly under cold water to remove any excess starch.
2. In a medium-sized saucepan, combine the rinsed rice, whole milk, and cinnamon stick.
3. Place the saucepan over medium heat and bring the mixture to a gentle simmer. Stir the contents frequently to prevent sticking or burning.
4. Once the mixture is simmering, lower the heat to low and allow it to cook, stirring occasionally, for approximately 25-30 minutes. You'll know it's done when the rice becomes tender, and the mixture thickens to a creamy consistency.
5. Stir in the granulated sugar and salt, making sure to dissolve the sugar completely.
6. Let the rice pudding continue to cook for an additional 5-10 minutes while stirring occasionally to avoid sticking.
7. Remove the saucepan from the heat and add the vanilla extract, stirring it into the pudding.
8. Allow the rice pudding to cool down slightly before transferring it to individual serving dishes or a large bowl.
9. Refrigerate the pudding until it is completely chilled.
10. Just before serving, sprinkle ground cinnamon over the top of the pudding for a traditional and aromatic garnish.
11. Enjoy this delightful and comforting "Arroz con Leche" pudding during your holiday feast or any special occasion!

NEXT STEP

Thanks for purchasing this book, reading it, and taking obedient action as you reflect on your food experiences & relationships. I hope it was enlightening and encouraging and that your life flourishes, one small step and one week at a time.

As you connect with more people & your lifestyle becomes healthier, you will influence many others around you, just like my friends in college influenced me unique food experiences that led me to create this book.

I would love to hear from you about how this book has impacted you. Your feedback
will help me in improving this book and other books in the future.

Receiving your review is important to me, it will help this book reach more people and change lives around the world.

www.ingramcontent.com/pod-product-compliance
Lightning Source LLC
Chambersburg PA
CBHW081443070526
44586CB00019B/2212